Culturally Diverse Populations: Reflections from Pioneers in Education and Research

The purpose of this book is to open a discourse on current and pertinent issues related to multicultural populations by the most noted experts and researchers in the field. This book offers an overview of the literature on multicultural populations and assesses its approach to a great variety of issues, including: ethnic sensitive practice, the diversity within multicultural populations, the teaching of diversity content, stereotypic assumptions with regard to filial piety and Asian American populations, substance abuse within the Latino community, multicultural youth and elders, refugee and immigrant populations as well as vulnerable populations such as victims of political and sexual exploitation. A broad spectrum of structural issues are also examined with regard to their impact on clients, the authors, and the community.

The aim is to provide a forum for educators in the field to present views regarding important issues for which there is no other venue. They are important for educators, practitioners, and students in the field to consider and discuss. These will serve as springboards for such discussion. Although references will be cited when appropriate, these will be position papers rather than research papers or reviews of the literature.

This book was based on a special issue of the *Journal of Ethnic and Cultural Diversity in Social Work*.

Diane de Anda is Professor Emerita in the Department of Social Welfare at the UCLA School of Public Policy and Social Research. Her most recent books are entitled *Violence: Diverse Populations and Communities* and *Social Work with Multicultural Youth*.

Culturally Diverse Populations: Reflections from Pioneers in Education and Research

Edited by Diane de Anda

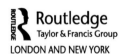

Routledge
Taylor & Francis Group

LONDON AND NEW YORK

First published 2009 by Routledge
2 Park Square, Milton Park, Abingdon, Oxon, OX14 4RN

Simultaneously published in the USA and Canada
by Routledge
270 Madison Avenue, New York, NY 10016

Routledge is an imprint of the Taylor & Francis Group, an informa business

© 2009 Edited by Diane de Anda

Typeset in Times by Value Chain, India
Printed and bound in Great Britain by CPI Antony Rowe, Chippenham, Wiltshire

British Library Cataloguing in Publication Data
A catalogue record for this book is available from the British Library

ISBN10: 0-7890-3197-3 (h/b)
ISBN10: 0-7890-3198-1 (p/b)
ISBN13: 978-0-7890-3197-6 (h/b)
ISBN13: 978-0-7890-3198-3 (p/b)

CONTENTS

Introduction:
Reflections from Pioneers
in Education and Research
on Culturally Diverse Populations

Diane de Anda

What follows is not the usual academic discourse. The aim of this collection of essays is to provide a venue for sharing reflections on topics of particular importance to the authors, who have been pioneers in developing the literature on multicultural populations in social work, the social sciences, education, public health, and related fields. Each was invited to contribute a thought-piece that would share their unique perspectives and conceptualizations, acquired over years of teaching, research, practice, and personal experience. Their essays integrate these varied sources of knowledge to elucidate a broad spectrum of issues.

Because I wished the collection to represent the unique voices of the authors rather than an editor's particular vision, the directive provided to the authors was broad. They were given complete latitude except that the manuscript was to be an essay rather than empirical research, that references to the literature were at their discretion as the main aim was to present their own voice, that the length could vary as they saw fit beyond a general guideline, and that the style in which they presented their reflections could be whatever they felt appropriate to their presentation.

As a result, the essays are marked by diversity in every respect, by the diverse populations of concern, by the wide range of issues that are addressed, by the style of presentation which varies from formal to case examples and personal memoirs, and by length which varies considerably by the scope of the topic and the style of presentation. What emerges is a sense of the rich bases of knowledge from which the expertise of the authors arises. What is also clear is that conceptualizations of issues related to culturally diverse populations have matured beyond general, homogeneous, descriptive accounts to a recognition of the great diversity within populations to which the profession must attend and the increasingly varied issues that must be addressed in serving these populations. The authors' presentations clearly demonstrate that serving our clients, be it through direct practice, research, policy, or advocacy, has become a more complex endeavor that requires new conceptualizations to which they lend their expertise. E-mail addresses have been provided for all authors with the hope that the essays will encourage dialogue and expand the discourse.

REFLECTIONS ON PRACTICE
AND RESEARCH
WITH MULTICULTURAL POPULATIONS:
PAST, PRESENT, AND BEYOND

Ethnic Sensitive Social Work Practice: Back to the Future

Elfriede G. Schlesinger
Wynetta Devore

INTRODUCTION

We begin this article with a great deal of excitement. It is a singular honor to have been asked to reflect on ethnic sensitive social work practice, how our work first developed, how it has evolved, and our perspective on the future.

Before we begin this overview, we would like to review the process that has led us to this point in our social work careers. We were both junior faculty at the School of Social Work at Rutgers University, one of us an African American woman, the other a Jewish American woman with some roots in the Holocaust. We had been teaching together, introducing content on race and class and ethnicity into the curriculum, and experimenting with a variety of ways to teach this perplexing material (Devore & Schlesinger, 1977).

There was limited literature on which to draw. Social work had paid virtually no attention to how ethnicity and social class issues were to be incorporated into practice. Importantly, some African American and Latino students thought the literature focused primarily on the presumed pathology of people of color. And so we began to write and do our own research (Schlesinger & Devore, 1977).

We talked about what it felt like to be African American, mothers, atheist, cultural Jew and refugee from the Holocaust, and committed Christian. Sometimes we clashed, but more often we agreed.

There was no doubt in our minds–based on personal, practice, and teaching experience as well as knowledge of the literature–that ethnicity affects our sense of ourselves, contributes to a sense of cohesion and sometimes to conflict. The importance of social class was also self-evident. While both of us had grown up poor, we were now thoroughly ensconced in the middle class and knew the difference well. Both positions have affected much of who we are as individuals.

From this it followed that ethnicity and social class affect those aspects of life with which social workers deal. It was out of these experiences and thinking that the major ideas presented in our work evolved.

It has been more than twenty-five years since the first edition of *Ethnic Sensitive Social Work Practice* was published (Devore & Schlesinger, 1981). When the original galleys were on display at the Annual Program Meeting of the Council on Social Work Education in Louisville, Kentucky in 1981, people stopped to look, to peek, and gave us the impression that the time for a work of this nature had come. The first formal review in *Social Work* supported that view (Chestang, 1982). Within the first few months of the book's publication, "ethnic sensitive" seemed to have become a part of our professional lexicon. Over the years, we applied the basic concepts to work on the family (Devore, 1983), to health care (Devore & Schlesinger, 1981), to Black/Jewish Relations (Schlesinger & Devore, 2001), and to new immigrants (Schlesinger & Devore, 2006).

For us, the basic concept is really quite simple. We essentially present the view that ethnicity and social class are key aspects of social functioning that need to be understood by social workers and incorporated into practice. Twenty-six years later we are pleased that most of the ideas originally presented remain viable. It is our view that we are all ethnics–no matter what the group. We have drawn on classic sociological literature on ethnicity and social class to develop our themes (e.g., Gordon, 1964).

Because racism and oppression of people of color were major aspects of American life–and still remain virulent–we have continued to stress social work's obligation to act to minimize oppression of all people. That people of color are especially oppressed in this country is a theme that recurs throughout our work. The effects of the major political and social movements of the sixties and seventies for civil rights, for women's rights, for gay rights and others informed our early work. These were underway then and are still in process.

Certainly we were not sufficiently prescient to foresee the dramatic developments that this country and the rest of the world would experience within the next twenty-five years. Particularly, we recognize the many demographic changes that were generated in large part by 1965 changes in immigration laws that revised entrenched policy that had limited entry to preferred European groups.

The world is a significantly different place now than when we first began our work. Yet, unfortunately, many of the problems we identified then remain with us. This overview examines some of the changes that inevitably affect our thinking. We try to capture the dynamic between continuity and change and the shape of ethnic sensitive practice of the future.

Our discussion begins with the presentation of a series of concepts that are key to our work. Some of these concepts are used frequently in the literature, but the several meanings often differ.

The "Changing Demographic Landscape" is presented next, highlighting the diversity of our changing population. This is followed by a discussion of ethnic identity and then "becoming part of American society," language we prefer to the classic notion of "assimilation" which has come under considerable scrutiny. Next we present an overview about the new immigrants. We discuss the "ethnic reality" and its implication for practice. We finish the paper with closing comments, examining whether our conceptualization and focus on the ethnic reality is still relevant for social work practice and education today.

ETHNIC SENSITIVE SOCIAL WORK PRACTICE: BASIC CONCEPTS AND RELATED DEFINITIONS

Culture is a frequently used word, with many meanings. Out of the many definitions we have studied, we use the term as a broad, overriding concept that revolves around the view that human groups differ in the way they structure their behavior, in their world view, in their perspectives on the rhythms and patterns of life, and how they perceive the essential nature of the human condition on matters such as the relationship between humans, the spirits, and the Gods (Devore & Schlesinger, 1999).

Some use the term culture to refer to different groups, as if they are "cultures." Others equate the term with ethnicity or ethnic groups. We make a clear distinction between ethnic groups and ethnicity and broad, overriding cultural themes.

Ethnic Groups. The basic view of ethnic groups developed in mid-20th century remains relevant. Some common themes converge: that ethnic groups share a common set of beliefs, common history, common religion, often similar physical features, a common language or some combination of these factors. Important is the view that the ethnic group serves as "a psychological referent" (Gordon, cited in Marger, 1996) and, importantly, that there is a sense of peoplehood. This affinity generates a comfort zone, when people congregate in their own groups.

Ethnic groups share a consciousness of kind, a sense of being like others and a sense of identity based on a shared history. Much of our daily life is in some ways impacted by the ethnic group, and how that group interprets universal events and fundamental cultural tenets. In today's world, people of different ethnic groups intermarry leading to ways people adapt and shift their sense of themselves.

It is our view that we are all ethnics, members of distinct groups, for example, Irish, Puerto Rican, or African American. Conceptually, we all share the features reviewed above. Given racism and oppression faced by many people of color, we have suggested (Devore & Schlesinger, 1999) that these groups–African Americans, Asian Americans, Latinos and Native Americans–be referred to as *oppressed ethnic groups*.

Race. We share the view held by many social scientists that race is a pejorative and destructive term, based on oppression and power issues, not on scientifically established biological distinctions between different peoples. The consequences of racial designations have long been destructive for too many people in this world.

Social Class is about inequality. The term refers to the horizontal stratification of the population related to economic life and to differences based on wealth, income, occupation, status, community power and other related matters. Commonly, in the United States, the population is divided into three or five levels. The most simple designation is upper, middle, and lower or working class. Position in the class structure is determined by the interaction between education, occupation and income. There is a considerable literature that suggests that many behaviors are a function of social class, including differences in achievement motivation, in perspectives on the importance of education, on gender issues as well as in matters of child rearing. The three social class variables in concert have considerable predictive power (Conley, 1999).

The Ethnic Reality. This concept was introduced early in our work and is the foundation of much of this work. The ethnic reality constitutes an integration of the person's experience of ethnicity and social class and the impact this has on all aspects of his/her life, including view of self and present and future opportunities. Its significance is discussed and illustrated in a later section of this paper.

THE CHANGING DEMOGRAPHIC LANDSCAPE

Overall Population Growth and Change

Between 1990 and 2000 the population of the United States grew by 13% or by 32.7 million people, the largest census to census increase in

American history (U.S. Census 2000; Community Survey, 2005); now, 10 years later, as of date of paper submission, August 7, 2007, at 17:57, the population of the United States was 302,544,804 (Census Clock, August 7, 2007).

Immigration is a key factor explaining this population growth, and continues apace. The increase in numbers of the population, together with the variety of immigrant ethnic groups, with their languages, their broad cultural precepts, and each with their unique coping styles, has had a profound impact on all of the American ways of life. Following is an overview of population statistics presenting a brief picture of current population distribution.[1]

African Americans are 12.1% of the population and Latinos, now the largest oppressed ethnic group, are at 14.6%. Asian Americans are 4.3% while Native Americans are under one percent (Census 2000: We the People: Asians in the United States, We the People: Hispanics in the United States). Oppressed ethnic groups constitute over 31% of our population. Less than 70% of the population is White. However, a view of these data for the nation as a whole does not tell the whole story. Many cities have lost considerable segments of their White population where more than half of the population is non-White. Overall, the top 100 cities saw a net reduction in the non-Hispanic White population of 2.3 million. The five largest cities lost nearly 1 million White residents. Growth of the Hispanic population was dramatic in most cities, a 43% increase over 1990 levels (Brookings Institution Center, 2001).

The census also asks a sample of the population to list the ancestry group with which they identify. Ancestry data are available for all groups, and the only extensive source of information in the census about the background of the White population. How much meaning their ancestry has for the White ethnics, or whether they have thoroughly assimilated into some "core" culture is in dispute, and is a matter to which we return later in this work. The five largest European ancestry groups listed in descending order are German, Irish, English, Italian and Polish (Ancestry, 2000). One group, Jewish people, is not covered in the census, because it is considered a religious group, although in our view it also qualifies as an ethnic group. As of 2004, there were around six million Jewish people in the United States (http://buff/c052302.htm). Between 1990 and 2000, there was a 20% decline in the three largest European ancestry groups–German, Irish and English. Nevertheless, there is a continuing migration from European countries; they are now 9.6% of the total number of new immigrants (Census 2000, Ancestry).

Populations of increasing interest, though small in number, are Arabs. Census 2000 reported that there were 850,000 people of Arab ancestry, including people from Lebanon, Egypt, Syria, Iraq, Morocco and others (Census 2000: We the People of Arab Ancestry in the United States, 2000).

Ethnic Identity

Ethnic identity essentially involves a sense of belonging. Important is the psychological attachment to the group. Citing Coleman and Rainwater (1978), Waters (1990) suggests that ethnicity adds spice to life in a postindustrial world; in a highly mobile population ethnic identity is important to people because it gives them a sense of heritage and roots.

As we go about our lives–as women and men, significant others, children, parents, workers–we approach life from some sense of who we are at core, a part of which is ethnic identity. For some, whether to share that identity is a matter of choice. People of color, whose identity is clearly visible, often sense subtle or direct negative responses to who they are. Intergroup tensions can surface subtly and intrude on the primary interaction. If we have learned to appreciate others and ourselves, our respective identities with their commonalities and differences can heighten the interaction.

Where the implicit or explicit answer to the question "Who am I"? is couched in terms of ethnic identity, many facets of life are likely to follow. Often it is pride in the group. When one is a member of a marginalized group, pride and anger may be intertwined. Many in this situation have experienced positive or negative, hurtful or embracing responses.

Ethnic identity is an important component of development. The 1950 work of Eric H. Erikson describes a time during which a developing person must establish a "sense of personal identity." Ethnic identity is an important component of personal identity. For second generation immigrant adolescents, there are a variety of identities available: to be an "American," a hyphenated American (e.g., Cambodian-American), a national origin person (e.g., Jamaican), or a panethnic identity (e.g., Latino, Asian). The adaptation of an ethnic identity and the establishment of ethnic loyalties may influence behavior and an outlook independent of the family's status (Rumbaut, 1996).

As children become more aware of their ethnic identity, they are likely to experience racial and ethnic discrimination. Each group is able to report experiences of discrimination and unfair treatment. Adolescents, who have such experiences, may develop incidents of depression and a pessimistic attitude. Still, there are others, though aware of discrimination related to the complexion of their skin, are able to affirm the belief in the promise of equality and claim their future as citizens of the United States.

As children from other countries settle here in the United States, the question of an ethnic identity looms large and may be confusing. There may be parental pressure to retain the "old ways," including retention of the native language, staying within the ethnic community, and engaging in familiar behaviors. At the same time, as they are trying to develop a sense of self that includes the habits and customs of this country, parental pressure appears to stand in their way. It becomes important to help families to find ways to retain pride in ongoing traditions while allowing the young people to move forward in the new country. In this respect the issues move beyond the formal declaration of being an American or a hyphenated American; they become part and parcel of the daily pulsing of life as people move within the family and between the family and the outer world. Recent studies serve to support this aspect of the development of an ethnic identity for many young people in immigrant families (e.g., Germain & Lien, 2005).

Zhou and Xiong (2005) have reviewed data from "The Second Generation and the Children of Immigrants Longitudinal Study" pertaining to how the Asians in the study identified themselves. Virtually none of the people in their 20's identified as unhyphenated Americans with the exception of some Japanese who were likely already in the third or fourth generation. Most identified as hyphenated Americans. To declare oneself as an unhyphenated American would also mean one identified as "White" since many of this group equate America with whiteness. This is true for many, including those who are fairly well acculturated, intermarry, and work hard toward gaining privileged middle class status.

Color, complexion, texture of hair, and facial features are declarations of membership in many oppressed ethnic groups. Patton (2006) explores self-image and racial identity in the lives of African American women and their struggles with beauty, body image, and hair. She suggests that for these women, having a White standard of beauty continually placed before them has often been destructive to the development of clear identity as a dark woman with an African heritage.

Members of White ethnic groups have choices in claiming an ethnic identity that is seldom available to persons of color. Although there is little question that there is a seeming comfort of membership in White ethnic groups, stereotypes persist. For example, a coalition of Italian

American organizations in Illinois filed a suit against a school board that permitted the presentation of a play that depicted Italians as uneducated and as mobsters (DeSantis, 2007). The highly successful film "My Big Fat Greek Wedding" has offended some Greek Americans, because it fails to break perceptions of Greek Americans as painting contractors and café owners. In either instance, affirmation of pride in ethnic identity has been called into question. However, negative images about a group can also reinforce ethnic identity. The effects may be to increase people's resolve to strengthen themselves and their group. Unfortunately, for some people, the onslaught of negative messages can be devastating.

Families will go to great length to provide experiences for their children which they hope will reinforce and strengthen children's ethnic identities. European ethnics have long sent their children to Hebrew School, and others, including new immigrant groups such as Ukrainians, to schools where the native language and customs are taught (Devore & Schlesinger, 1999), reinforcing the ethnic identity transmitted through the family, religious, and other ethnic institutions, including ethnic based social services that have long been developed as a way of reaching out to "one's own."

As social workers work with people, we try to help them to draw on their ethnic identity as a source of strength highlighting the group's resources as a way of dealing with the problems.

Intermarriage and Ethnic Identity

Marriage to a person not of one's group, an increasingly common experience in this country, inevitably has an effect on people's ethnic identity. Engaging in one of the world's most intimate relationship with a person who does not share one's ethnic identity almost inevitably involves some rethinking of the degree of commitment to one's own group. Further, many families, often even those from whom one would least expect it, cast a jaundiced eye on the prospect. The extent to which such marriages may involve differences in religious observances, how holidays are spent, and related matters can affect daily life. Perlman and Waters (2007) suggest that "intermarriage has played havoc with simple definitions of ethnic origin and generation by the time the grandchildren of the immigrants come of age" (p. 111). Intermarriage clearly generates multiple identities with major consequences for the way we think about ourselves and our interaction with other people. Studies of intermarriage look at how often people cross the boundaries of the broad racial groups to form couples, the ultimate consequence of an increasingly diverse society.

BECOMING PART OF AMERICAN SOCIETY

During the planning of this work, we determined that there would be a portion with a particular focus on "assimilation" given the importance of immigration at the beginning of the 21st century. Assimilation is what we who think and write about ethnicity have long called the process by which newcomers make their way in this country. However, based on a review of some of the important current thought on the subject, we came to the conclusion that perhaps the concept of assimilation was not the only, nor perhaps the best way to think about this subject, a point made by Alba and Nee (2007). They point out that many people view the term as "an ethnocentric and patronizing imposition on the minority people struggling to retain their cultural and ethnic integrity" (p. 124).

The pre-1965 history of immigration–its trials and its joys–has been told by us and others (Devore & Schlesinger, 1999). Our focus here is on the present group of immigrants, and what the experience of the earlier groups can tell us about the newcomers.

Much of the discussion of "assimilation" has focused on whether and how newcomers come to participate in the economic mainstream, whether they speak English, and to what extent they adopt the main customs of the society. Questions persist as to whether ethnic identity persists well past the point of initial adaptation, including into the second and subsequent generations.

Persistence of Ethnicity

A major area of continuing interest has focused on the persistence of ethnicity, and whether and to what extent immigrants retain a sense of identity with their original ethnic groups. Much study has been centered on whether second and subsequent generations retain command of the native language, whether they identify with the group's customs and values, whether they tend to intermarry or marry out of their native group, and how involved they are in carrying out ethnic rituals, such as customary holiday celebration.

Analysts focusing on the experience of the post-1965 immigrants have been looking at what happened to the European ethnics as a way of understanding what is likely to happen to the current group of newcomers.

When we reviewed the literature on the persistence of ethnicity among Europeans, it seemed that there were two worlds of scientific scholarship. One group of analysts has come to the conclusion that distinctive ethnic groups among the Europeans are a thing of the past (Hirschman, 1991). Another group takes the position that on the daily matters of life, as for example, when it comes to matters of mental health, ethnic group differences loom large.

Support for the view expressed by Hirschman (1991) comes from extensive intermarriage among European ethnics, the fact that few know the ethnic language or have ethnic political concerns, ". . . to put the matter simply, there is very little left of ethnicity for most white Americans" (p. 181).

Portes and Rumbaut (2005) share this view. They contend that children of European immigrants learned English, gradually abandoned their parents' language and "clawed their ways through schools and entrepreneurship into economic affluence . . . By the third generation, foreign languages were a distant memory and ethnic identities were social conveniences, displayed on selected occasions, but subordinate to overwhelming American selves" (pp. 985-986).

McGoldrick, Giordano, and Pearce (1996), who have studied the whole range of ethnic groups, suggest that ethnic groups differences become evident when people experience mental health problems and other life crises. In their view, many social science researchers have failed to realize that when European Americans who consider themselves to be fully assimilated experience periods of stress and personal difficulty, they often return to familiar sources of comfort, including ethnic rituals and behaviors. According to many authors included in their 1996 work, any number of examples of the retention of differences can be identified; there are those that have almost become part of the common lore: the overprotective Jewish mother, the stoic English, and the humor and pathos of the Irish. Our own review of work on European ethnics found throughout our work (e.g., Devore & Schlesinger, 1999) points to many areas of daily life where people draw on their ethnic background as they deal with life. These include responses to matters of physical as well as mental health, and to decision making around how to care for the elderly in their families.

In our view, ethnicity persists among European ethnics, precisely in the areas of social work concern, no matter whether they have achieved middle class status or have intermarried. People who are stoic in the face of pain pose different diagnostic challenges to physicians than those who are especially voluble. The same is true when a social worker is trying to assess whether a particular parent-child relationship is "pathologically enmeshed" or is characteristic of the customs of the ethnic group to which the clients belong. Our own personal experience, and that of the many students with whom we have worked over the years, supports the view of the persistence of ethnicity. Clearly, the degree of persistence varies for European ethnics as it does for any other group. Our task, as social workers, is to discern the impact of the difference in respect to the situation at hand.

Social Class and Race as Factors in Becoming Part of American Society

There are clear differences between the new immigrants and those of an earlier period. Major among these is the fact that most of the new immigrants are considered "racial and ethnic minorities," thus limiting the likelihood of full assimilation. Xie and Greenman (2007) in their analysis of segmented assimilation theory, outline several possible assimilation paths. One follows the traditional path into the middle class. The second is acculturation and assimilation into the urban underclass, resulting in poverty and downward mobility. In this group are those, like some Haitians, who, facing barriers to a comfortable life, become part of the seriously disadvantaged group of young Blacks.

A third involves purposeful preservation of the immigrant community's values (Xie & Greenman, 2007). This perspective is based on the fact that the United States is a highly stratified and unequal society. Given this, people will assimilate into different segments of the society. Fernandez-Kelly and Konczal (2005) put it this way: "social class plays a role in 'segmenting' the fate of children" (p. 1177). There are also those whose families have or develop resources, who remain immersed in the ethnic community, and have limited contact with groups other than their own. Foner and Kasinitz (2007) find that connections with the ethnic enclaves of the parents does not facilitate upward mobility. However, a strong connection can provide a safety net for those who are less successful.

It is clear, that the process long considered "assimilation" is no longer, if it ever was, a straight line into the middle class of White America. Analysts of considerable reputation have different points of view, each predicting different outcomes for the current groups of immigrants.

Waters and her colleagues (2004, 2007) have an essentially optimistic outlook, as do Alba and Nee (2007), although their views on the likely long range outcome differ. Despite their differences, all have found that the resources of the first generation have a major impact on the outcome of the second generation. When people come with few skills and limited if any education, the likelihood of a successful future for the next generation is worrisome. Foner and Kasinitz (2007) fear for the second generation of Mexican American immigrants. This group is large, and a high proportion of their parents have little education and work in low status occupations. They drop out of high school at high rates. Nevertheless, a large number do better in education and income than their parents.

From the perspective of ethnic sensitive practice, it is clear that the new immigrants, as well as substantial numbers of long resident people–Native Americans–face substantial problems, as well as growth and positive change.

The work of Portes and Rumbaut (2005) and that of Waters and her colleagues (2004) both explicitly and implicitly point to the role of social class in the lives of immigrants. Social class, together with the structure of beliefs and values of the various groups, have a significant impact on the second generation.

Becoming a part of American society is an ongoing process. In our view, as we have already stated, we are all ethnics. The degree to which ethnicity affects our daily life is a function of many complex, sometimes subtle, factors. It is too soon to dismiss ethnicity as a significant portion of the life of any individual or group.

THE NEW IMMIGRANTS

Here we refer essentially to the people who came to settle in this country following the 1965 changes in immigration policy. Our presentation is limited in scope and does not offer a complete description or analysis of the current group of newcomers. Rather, we present some key information about who the immigrants are, where they live, and some of their joys and sorrows as these have bearing on ethnic sensitive practice in the 21st Century

Undocumented immigrants have been coming to this country in large numbers. The Census does not ask the foreign born if they are legal residents. However, the Census and a variety of other organizations have drawn on census data to estimate the size of this population. By March 2005, there were about 9.8 million undocumented residents of whom around six million are working. It is estimated that the undocumented residents account for about one half of the recent growth in the immigrant population (Urban Institute, 2004).

Income

Different groups have been participating in the economy and the educational system, but at differing rates. Comparing Asian and Latino incomes, (Census 2000–We the People: Asians in the United States, We the People: Latinos in the United States) we find that compared to all workers in the United States who (had median earnings of $37,057), Asian workers have the highest incomes. As a whole the mean earnings of Asian men were, in 1999, $40,650 and $31,049 for women. Comparable figures for all Latinos are $25,400 and $21,634. However, there are major within group differences. Among Asians, the highest earning groups are Asian Indian men ($51,904) and Japanese men ($50,876). Among Latinos, the highest earning groups are Cuban men ($31,527) and Spanish men ($39,628).

In the same year (1999), the poverty rate for the total population was 12.4%, for the overall Asian population, 12.6%, and for the overall Latino population, 22.6%. Within group differences were substantial. Among Asian Americans, the highest poverty rate was among the Hmong at 37.8% and the lowest among the Japanese and Asian Indians (9.7% and 9.8%). The comparable data for Latinos are 25.8% for Puerto Ricans and 27.5% for Dominicans with the lowest among Cubans (14.6%) and Spaniards (12.8%).

Comparable data on education, looking only at people with a bachelors degree or better, are in the same vein. Of the total population, as of 1999, 24.4% had at least a bachelor's degree, as did 44.1% of Asians, and 10.4% of Latinos. The highest number of bachelor's degrees among Asians were earned by Asian Indians 63.9%, and among Latinos, by South Americans (25.2%) and Cubans (21.2%).

Looking at these figures it is very clear that both Latinos and Asians have generated social class structures comparable to those of the American population as a whole with substantial gaps between the upper middle class and those at the lower end of the class ladder. Any type of social work intervention needs to be attuned to these differences, and how their social class status together with their ethnic group impact on their lives.

Residential Patterns

More than ever before, immigrants are settling in many areas of the country. A walk, a trip to the market, a glimpse into our schools, reveals the growing diversity almost everywhere. Nevertheless, in keeping with a long standing pattern, the largest numbers of immigrants continue to live in the six states where many have been settling in this current cohort: California, New York, Texas, Florida, New Jersey and Illinois. Immigrants have long favored cities and metropolitan areas as places to live, and this remains the case at present.

At present, they are more likely to live in central cities, 44% of the foreign born compared to 27% of the native born. At present, the largest number of foreign born live in: New York, 35.9% of the population, Los Angeles 41%, Chicago 22%, Houston 26.4% and Miami, almost 60%. But the newcomers are also coming to areas of the country where people are less familiar with the new immigrants who are largely Asians and Latinos. One source reports that a number of these areas have seen substantial increases in immigrant populations over the past period: Indiana, 34%, South Dakota, 44%, Delaware, 32%, and New Hampshire, 26%. Actually, the list goes on. None of these data sources distinguish between documented and undocumented workers (The Brookings Institution Center on Urban and Metropolitan Policy, 2001).

What is clear, is that a growing number of the new immigrants are living and working in all areas of the country. In some states they have come to work in relatively small cities that were experiencing a declining economy as plants began to close, and, in effect, helped to bring the cities out of economic doldrums (Shared Histories, Shared Hopes, 2003).

A Brief Sketch of Immigrants Across the Country

Pictures of immigrants are seen daily in the media. We see images of "illegals" crossing the border into Arizona and New Mexico, and parents of American born children being deported, leaving the children without their families.

We find people who speak little English working in hotels and restaurants and as gardeners and construction workers. We also see those with a better command of the language working in banks and other occupations requiring higher skills. As social work educators, we see students from far and wide in our classes, some struggling with the language while preparing for a career in our profession. Some are planning to return to work in their homeland, others want to stay here.

As social work practitioners we see people with a range of problems, not unlike those we see with all people. Some are specific to their immigration status. If they are undocumented, they are always fearful.

We have already presented data on their earnings and education. Behind those figures lurk data on poverty, especially of children. Fass and

Cauthen (2006) report that 26% of immigrant children are poor, and that having an immigrant parent increases the chances of being poor. First generation immigrants constitute one-sixth of the population of the United States, and one-fourth of all poor people in the United States (Rector, 2006).

The impact of poverty is well-known to social workers and needs little comment here, except to say that poor children are always our special concern. Poverty is highly interrelated with poor education and poor health.

Second Generation Immigrants

Much of the work on becoming part of America to which we have already referred points out that it is the experience of the second generation and beyond that will tell the tale of how this group of immigrants is making adaptations to this country. Portes and Rumbaut (2005) suggest that the first generation simply sets the stage for the next generation. A group of second generation young New Yorkers studied by Kasinitz, Mollenkopf, and Waters (2004) are described as people whose parents were immigrants, but who themselves were born and raised in the United States. They view themselves as very different from their parents, with different educational experiences; they think about race and ethnicity differently from their parents and hold differing views in relation to love, marriage, and family relationships, viewing themselves as mainstream Americans daily balancing their ethnic heritage with their "Americaness." A series of studies in *Becoming New Yorkers* (2004) highlights the varied experiences of the range of Latino and Asian American second generation. The studies show, for the most part, that ethnic dispositions intersect with their parents social class disposition, and how they are received in this country to affect their fate as Americans.

Several of these studies highlight the differences between social classes within the same larger ethnic group. For example, Louie (2004) shows that pre-college age Chinese men and women, children of small entrepreneurs (restaurants, laundries), select public colleges in New York City, whereas those whose parents are highly educated "head for the ivies." The value placed on education in both class groups is similar. Young Koreans who have not been as successful as is expected, shy away from a Korean identity, because not to have succeeded is a failure in the eyes of other young Korean Americans (Lee, 2004). Rumbaut (1996) also considers the adaptive experiences of the second generation in a description of dissonant acculturation as the experience of growing up in a family when children learn English and American ways. The potential for a gap between language and other ethnic traditions is significant. Conflicts between generations become evident as children are embarrassed by adults who attempt to fit in with American peers. The stress of adolescence along with the need to adapt to the larger society are issues that are not uncommon in families of second-generation adolescents. These intergenerational relationships will be mediated within the family in relation to a variety of circumstances, including parent's socioeconomic position, family structure, peer networks as well as school context. As it may well be during adolescence of any ethnic group, there is the impact of interpersonal and intrapersonal relationships.

The One-and-a-Half (1.5) Generation

One-and-a-half (1.5) generation immigrants have been identified as young people who have spent their developmental years in the United States, but who were born in their parents' countries of origin. Their adaptation experiences are unlike those of second-generation youth or adult immigrants. Studies related to the experiences of 1.5 generation Koreans determined that these individuals have been able to operate proficiently within and between Korea and the United States environments. One-and-a-half generation people have been said to have high degrees of socialization in the United States and indigenous culture as well. In addition, this group will have fluency in English and their native language as well. Given this agility with language, this generation is called upon to serve as family "cultural brokers," responsible for translation in family and public matters. Respondents in the Kim, Brenner, Lang, and Asay (2003) study strongly identified with U.S. culture, trying to become as "Americanized" as possible, but at the same time reveled in the rich culture of their countries of origin in behaviors such as Filipino humility and respect for family and elders.

Instances of discrimination and racism were again experienced to varying degrees from friendliness in predominately White neighborhoods to being bullied by members of other ethnic groups, having teachers make racist remarks, being asked ignorant questions regarding ethnic stereotypes, or teasing related to accents. In addition there were reports of discrimination from members of their own ethnic groups. Still, they have been able to establish relationships with people from different ethnic groups (Kim, Brenner, Lang, & Asay, 2003).

Adding to the scant literature related to this population is an examination of the experiences of one-and-a-half generation Mexican youth who were students attending the University of Oregon (Gonzales-Berry, Mendoza, & Plaza, 2006). Their parents had entered the United States as undocumented workers who took agricultural jobs. Eventually they were able to become permanent residents. These students and other one-and-a-half generation children arrived speaking only Spanish. Soon they became bilingual, but their younger Spanish-speaking siblings soon became linked to English, abandoning their native language. This experience is much like that of second-generation children who are familiar with the language of their parents, but tend to speak English primarily.

Students recalled early experiences in the United States, where they discovered that "color" could be a burden added to a variety of experiences of structural discrimination in school with peers, faculty, and staff. Given our concern about childhood and adolescent development, we recognize the damage that such experiences may do as young people mature. Peers and older siblings whose negative experiences have left them disaffected may encourage behaviors that reject the values of family and community. However, again as in other immigrant groups, family and community offer support. Educational aspirations and expectations advocated by immigrants' parents might persist in spite of deterrents.

Like 1.5 generation Asian college students (Kim, Brenner, Lang, & Asay, 2003), these youth claim identity as Americans as well as Mexicans. They have no doubt that they belong to this country, having chosen the best of Mexico and the United States as they sculpted their own identities. One student's remarks may well synthesize the experience of many,

> I would like to live here, not in Mexico, because my family is here. I have relatives in Mexico there, but I have more security here. I feel that I don't belong there anymore. The experiences of my relatives in Mexico have been different from mine. I have more passion to fight against injustices here.

THE ETHNIC REALITY

The "ethnic reality" is a concept we first introduced in 1981 (Devore & Schlesinger, 1981). It is the conceptual base of the model of ethnic sensitive practice derived from sociological stratification theory. Derived from Gordon's discussion (1964) of "ethclass" as a way of thinking about the differences in outlook between people at the same social class level, but members of different ethnic groups, Gordon thought that social class is of primary importance as a determinant of the basic conditions of life, a perspective that we have shared and continue to share. The basic premise is that social class as an amalgam of education, occupation and income, as earlier described, in large measure determines our life chances. It affects what we can buy, where we can afford to live, where we can send our children to school, what kind of health care to which we have access, and importantly, the kind of work we do. These are all connected to the chances we have for a comfortable life or one of economic hardship and struggle.

As best as we can determine, we remain among the few, if any, analysts who focus on social class status as a way of thinking about various groups, whether White, people of color, or immigrants. Much more of the work of other analysis has focused on "culture." More recently, Fong touched on the intersect between culture and social class (Fong, 2004). As already pointed out, analysis of post-1965 immigrants has begun to focus on social class. For example, Fernandez–Kelly and Konczal (2005) suggests that social class most broadly determines personal and collective options. They view class, ethnicity, and race as overlapping; identities are formed along these dimensions and are considered cultural capital which contribute to group identity.

Each ethnic and class configuration of the various groups, taken together, highlights key features of social life and begins to explain both commonality and variation between the groups.

These configurations and the cluster of outlooks they represent variously reflect perspectives on matters ranging from political outlook to views on child rearing, to features of family life, and responses to health and illness. At the same time, people who continue to believe in some of the traditional views on the cause and treatment of illness–people still immersed in traditional belief systems–will differ from those socialized to Western traditions.

We have used the "ethnic reality" to analyze key features of life as they bear on ethnicity and social class and related concepts. For example, over the years we have analyzed the similarities and differences between African Americans at various points on the class structure, highlighting how common oppression can join those who have benefited economically from life in the United States to those at the lower rungs; both are suffering from racism. Reference has also been made to the situation of American Indians who feel a tension between what they are expected to do at work as members of the American work force, as people who reside on a social class stratum, and with regard to obligations to family, so deeply ingrained in American Indian ethnic dispositions.

Today it is said that American Jews are largely middle class. Yet, data show that there are poor Jewish people, especially among the elderly and more recent Jewish immigrants from Russia (National Jewish Population Survey, 2007). Here too, the impact of group expectations clash with individual economic realities. In contrast, some young African Americans have developed the view that to do well in school and rise in the class structure is in conflict with being loyal to one's group. For some, these are powerful beliefs, which they believe are essential to the maintenance of their group; in turn, these beliefs hold some back from developing the knowledge and skills expected in this society.

Most recently (Schlesinger & Devore, 2006), we analyzed the situation of Asian and Latino Americans, many of them fairly recent immigrants, to determine whether the concepts embedded in the "ethnic reality" were useful to understand their lives. We found that Asians as a whole and Latinos as a whole, are distributed along the American social class structure in a fashion characteristic of all the people of the United States.

Earlier, in the discussion of the new immigrants, we presented key income and education figures, as well as class distribution for Latino and Asian populations. In analyzing the experiences of some Asian and Latino groups, the Asian Indians and Hmong among the Asians, and Dominicans and Cubans among the Latinos, it became clear that reference to the broad Asian and Latino cultural perspectives were not sufficient to understand their specific experiences as immigrants. Rather, the concept of the ethnic reality, and its focus, the convergence of social class and ethnicity, is more useful because it allows us to integrate their long standing cultural and ethnic precepts with their current social class status. Asian Indians are among the best educated and have the best incomes of all of these groups. Many of the Asian Indian immigrants were sought after by the United States when this country found itself in need of people with high level technological and other professional skills.

These Asian Indians have been able to achieve without giving up many of their ethnic dispositions. Many maintain the custom of wearing traditional clothing, of parental selection of a spouse for their children, and extensive, ongoing involvement with the extended family, community and religion (from U.S. Census Press Releases http://www.census.gov/Press-release/www/releases/archives/facts_for_features_special_e; Lal, 2007). The Hmong, by contrast, fled from their country after having little choice but to participate in the war in Laos in the 1960's and early 1970's. They are a very rural people; many on first arrival illiterate in their own language have no ability to understand or speak English. In addition, they have been found to be very much immersed in their own religious practices (History and Culture of the Hmong People, 2006). As the years since their initial migration have increased, many more Hmong are becoming integrated into the lives of their communities; however, for some it is difficult to give up the old ties (Davey, 2007).

Dominicans, among the lowest paid and least educated of the Latino groups, have come as migrant laborers, carrying out poorly paid, low status work. They share the behavior of many immigrants, of leaving their country with the hope that they will be able to bring their families to the United States or of returning home for a more comfortable life. Unfortunately, too often they did not find a welcome. Lopez's (2004) study of a New York City High School where many Dominican students are enrolled, depicts the school as dilapidated, badly maintained, and little optimism among students or their teachers about their educability.

By contrast, many Cubans, especially those who escaped from the Castro regime were welcomed and resources were made available. Unlike their Dominican peers, many were highly educated or experienced in business when they arrived. They soon formed close communities, especially in Florida, which served as high level supports. Fernandez-Kelly and Konczal (2005) cite the experiences of several groups of Cubans in Florida, where the class position of the family interacts with the reception received in the United States to shape the lives of the second generation. They believe, as we do that "social class most broadly determines personal and collective options" (p. 1157).

It seemed to us, that this mode of analysis as a way of explaining the lives of different groups allows us to see that ethnically-based dispositions come to play in daily life and interact with social class and its impact on life. The Asian Indians and the Hmong both derive their basic cultural precepts from Asian culture: its view of people to people relationship and the importance of incorporating the gods and spirits into one's life. However, the Asian Indian and the Hmong experience, both before migration and life in the United States are much more affected by the more current ethnic and class dispositions. Each group has a different set of religious beliefs and different access to education, matters that ultimately determine how they will fare in this country.

In our teaching, we have also used the "ethnic reality" as a way of analyzing case material and assessing how class and ethnicity are shaping and contributing to the problems about which they are seeing the social worker. Social class, as a factor explaining the lives of the people seen by social workers, has been sorely neglected in our literature and in our practice. Ethnicity, or sometimes culture, without reference to social class does not focus sufficiently on how these factors work together to affect our lives. For these and related reasons we believe that "the ethnic reality" is a useful analytic concept.

CLOSING COMMENTS

We began this paper by pointing to the dramatic changes that have taken place in this country since we first began our work, more than 25 years ago. In these closing comments then, a major question for us is whether these changes have been of such a nature as to require major re-formulation or recasting of our work.

Our major impetus for writing *Ethnic Sensitive Social Work Practice* was that social work, both in practice and education, had paid insufficient attention to ethnicity and social class. Although there were a number of works that did address related issues, there was virtually nothing that dealt with the integration of this type of understanding into practice; rather, there had been a tendency to consider these matters as background material, important to know, but not really to use.

Much has changed in this respect. There is a growing, rich literature, and related content is a required part of social work education. A lot of this work differs from ours in many respects. Major among these differences is our emphasis on social class as an important factor in life, especially when it is integrated with understanding of people's ethnic group membership.

Our review of various theories of assimilation has shown that indeed social class plays a major factor in the lives of the newcomers. With few exceptions, analysts who differ in other respects make this point. The socioeconomic starting place of the first generation, whether of low skill, limited economic resources and education, or considerable social capital and middle class status, have major impact on the subsequent generation.

Zhou and Xiong (2005) highlight the impact of racism on the new immigrants. Those who are in the lower class groups are only minimally protected by their ethnically and culturally-honed coping styles. Like the rest of the society, they are caught in the travails of a racist, capitalist society.

Present and future immigrants, especially the undocumented, are under assault. As they function in a society that is so ambivalent about their presence, a layer of fear is added to their ongoing effort to become a part of America. We have all seen and heard about the raids on their homes and places of work, sometimes sweeping those with green cards in the net. Social work has a special obligation to advocate for and protect this group of people, and the contribution they make to this country.

Also relatively unique and different from other social work analysts is our view that "we are all ethnics." Much of the other literature focuses on what we call oppressed ethnic groups, virtually having wiped "off the map" European Americans and other groups that don't neatly fit into this categorization. Indeed, many who have been more than complimentary about our work have the impression that we are all about "minority" issues.

This has been troublesome for us in many ways. As our discussion has shown, about 70% of Americans are White, a significant number of them are members of the working class and are poor, and many have the types of problems that bring them to social workers. For the past twenty plus years, we have not been educating our students for practice with a large number of Americans. Our accreditation requirements have appropriately stressed vulnerable populations, but have excluded so many of them.

From an ideological point of view, this exclusion if you will, of White populations from our syllabi and our literature has created a "we-them" situation between students of color and all others. For White students, it subtly reinforced a sense of superiority, for it was "them" not me, who needed to be understood.

As our population has become more diverse, it is more necessary than ever to take the view that we are all ethnics, or all people, whose lives need to be understood if social workers are to be effective. The list of the American people is long; we need to find a way of educating ourselves about them, without making lists of who is in, and who is out.

We located ethnic sensitive practice within the broader framework of practice theories and interventive approaches, all the while suggesting how long-honed practice knowledge and skill need to be adapted to the ethnic- and class-based beliefs and habits of the people with whom we work. Since we began, there has been much rich work done on the strengths and empowerment perspectives. We were most pleased when some of the people who worked on these new perspectives suggested that our work had contributed the groundwork needed to move in this direction (Lee, 2001). We have much to learn from these approaches and look forward to incorporating their themes in our own work.

In answer to our own question as to whether our work needs fundamental reformulation and restructuring, we immodestly say no. We have paid a lot of attention in this paper to the new immigrants, because it is imperative that social workers understand this population. This highly focused look has helped to highlight key features of our perspective. For us, the concept of the ethnic reality has reinforced the importance of social class in American society. We will continue to address the concerns of all people–recognizing the special concerns of oppressed ethnic groups.

NOTE

1. The major source for these data are various documents from the United States Census 2000 and population estimates of the 2005 American Community Survey.

REFERENCES

Alba, R. & Nee, R. (2007). Assimilation. In Waters, M. C. & R. Ueda. *The New Americans.* Cambridge, MA. Harvard University Press.
——————-(2003). *Remaking the American Mainstream.* Cambridge, MA. Harvard University Press.
Chestang, L. (1982). Book Reviews: Shirley Jenkins, The ethnic dilemma in social services and Wynetta Devore and Elfriede G. Schlesinger, Ethnic sensitive social work practice. *Social Work, 27,* 117.
Coleman, R. P. (1978). *Social standing in America: New dimensions in social class.* New York: Basic Books.
Conley, D. (1999). *Being Black, living in the red.* Berkely, California: University of California Press.
Davey, M. (2007). Leader's arrest uncovers divide in Hmong-Americans. *The New York Times.* Thursday, June 14. A20
DeSantis, D. (2007). Coalition to sue school officials for stereotyping Italian Americans. Washington: Italian Americans. Vol. 12, 1(3).
Devore, W. (1983). The ethnic reality and work with Black families. *Social Casework, 64,* 525-531.
Devore, W. & Schlesinger, G. (1977). The integration of social science and literary materials: An approach to teaching urban family life. *Journal of Education for Social Work, 1*(3), 12-18.
Devore, W. & Schlesinger, E. (1981). *Ethnic sensitive social work practice.* New York: Merrill.

Devore, W. & Schlesinger E. (1987). *Ethnic sensitive social work practice.* 2nd Edition 2. Columbus, Ohio: Merrill.

Devore, W. & Schlesinger, E. (1991). *Ethnic sensitive social work practice.* 3rd Edition. New York: Merrill.

Devore, W. & Schlesinger, E. (1995). *Ethnic sensitive social work practice.* 4th Edition. Boston: Allyn & Bacon.

Devore, W. & Schlesinger, E. (1999). *Ethnic sensitive social work practice.* 5th Edition. Boston: Allyn & Bacon.

Devore, W. & Schlesinger, E. (1977). The integration of social science and literary materials: An approach to teaching urban family life. *Journal of Education for Social Work,* (*1*) 3.

Erickson, E. (1950). *Childhood and society.* New York: Norton.

Falk, G. *American Jews.* http://www.buff.com/c 052302.htm. Downloaded August 6, 2007.

Fass, S. & Cauthen, G. (2006). Who are America's poor children? *National Center for Children in Poverty.* http://www.org/publications/show.php?id_684. Downloaded August 6, 2007.

Fernandes-Kelly, P. & Konczal, L. (2005). Murdering the alphabet: Identity and entrepreneurship among second-generation Cubans, West Indians and Central Americans. *Ethnic and Racial Studies, 28*(6), 1153-1181.

Fix, M. & Capps, R. (2005). Immigrant children, urban schools and the No Child Left Behind Act. http://www.Migrationinformation.org/Feature/display.cfm?id=347. Downloaded August 6, 2007.

Fong, R. (2004). *Culturally competent practice with immigrant and refugee children and families.* New York: Guilford Press.

Gans, H. (1979). Symbolic ethnicity: The future of ethnic groups and cultures in America. *Ethnic and Racial Studies, 28*(6), 1151-1181.

Gordon, M. (1964). *Assimilation in American life: The role of race, religion and national origins.* New York: Oxford University Press.

Germine, R. & Lien, J. H. (2005). Ego Identity and the Psychosocial well being of ethnic minority and majority college students. *Lea on Line.* http://www.leasonline.com/do. Downloaded August 6th, 2007.

Gonzales-Berry, E., Mendoze, M., & Plaza, D. (2006). One-and-a-half generation Mexican youth in Oregon: Pursuing the mobility dream. Oregon State University Department of Ethnic Studies.

Hirschman, C. (1991). What happened to the white ethnics? *Contemporary Sociology, 20*(2), 180-183.

History and Culture of the Hmong People (2006). http://www.uwex.edu/ces/wnep/hmong/bckgrd.htm. Downloaded February, 10, 2006.

Johnson, L. A. (2006). Documentary, studies renew debate about skin color's impact. *Pittsburg Post-Gazette.* December 26.

Kasinitz, P. Mollenkopf, J. H., & Waters, M. C. (2004). *Becoming New Yorkers; Ethnographies of the second generation.* New York: Russell Sage Foundation.

Kim, B. S., Brenner, B. R., & Asay, P. A. (2003). *Cultural diversity and ethnic minority psychology, 9*(2), 156-170.

Lee, J. A. B. (2001). *The empowerment approach to social work practice.* New York: Columbia University Press.

Lee, S. (2004). Class matters, racial and ethnic identities of working and middle-class second generation Korean Americans. In P. Kasinitz, J. H. Mollenkopf, & M. C. Waters, Eds., *Becoming New Yorkers*. New York: Russell Sage Foundation.

Louie, V. (2004). "Being practical" or "Doing what I want," The role of parents in the academic choices of Chinese Americans. In P. Kasinitz, J. H. Mollenkopf, & M. C. Waters, Eds., *Becoming New Yorkers*. New York: Russell Sage Foundation.

Marger, M. N. (1997). *Race and ethnic relations*. Belmon, CA: Wadsworth.

McGoldrick, M., Gordans, J., & Pearce, J. K. (1996). *Ethnicity and family therapy.* New York: The Guilford Press.

Patton, T. C. (2006). Hey girl, am I more than my hair? African American women and their struggles with beauty, body image and hair. *NWSA Journal.* Summer *18*(2), 24-28.

Paral, R. (2006). The growth and reach of immigration. *Policy Brief.* http://www.allf. org/ipc/policybrief/policybrief_2006_81606.shtml

Perlman, J. & Waters, M. C. (2007). Intermarriage and multiple identities. In *The New Americans: A Guide to Immigration Since 1965.* Cambridge, Mass: Harvard University Press.

Portes, A. & Rumbaut, R. G. (1996). *Immigrant American: A portrait.* 2nd Edition. Berkely, CA: University of California Press.

—————————(2005). Introduction: The second generation and the children of immigrants longitudinal study. *Ethnic and Racial Studies, 6,* 985-999.

Rector, R. E. (2006). *Importing poverty: Immigration and poverty in the United States: A book of charts.* http://www.heritage.org/wherewent. Downloaded August 6, 2007.

Schlesinger, E. G. & Devore, W. (1979). Social workers view ethnic minority teaching. *Journal of Education for Social Work. 15*(3), 20-27.

Schlesinger, E. G. and Devore, W. (1981). Social work practice in health care: An ethnic sensitive approach. *Journal of Sociology and Social Welfare, VIII* (4), 858-876.

Schlesinger, Elfriede G., & Devore, W. (2001). African Americans and Jewish Americans; Searching for a new song. *New Global development: Journal of International and Comparative Social Welfare, XVII.* (1&2), 63-73.

Schlesinger, E. G. & Devore, W. (2006). A return to ethnicity and social class; The immigration experience. A Paper Presented at the Annual Meeting of the Council on Social Work Education: Chicago, Illinois. February.

Shared history, shared hopes: A photo exhibit: Documenting the contributing struggles and dreams of Idaho's immigrant communities. (2003). http://www.nwfco.org/ 08-28-03 Shared History Shared Hopes. Dowloaded August 7, 2007.

The Brookings Center on Urban and Metropolitan Policy. (2001). Racial and ethnic change in the nation's largest cities: Evidence from the 2000 Census. http://www.brook.edu/es/urban/census/citygrowth.htm. Downloaded July 10, 2007.

United States Census: 2000

United States Census: Community Survey, 2005

United States Census 2000: Ancestry 2000

United States Census 2000: We the People: Hispanics in the United States

United States Census 2000: We the People: Asians in the United States

United States Census 2000: We the People: We the People of Arab Ancestry in the United States

United States Census Clock, August 7, 2007

Waters, Mary, C. (1990). *Ethnic options: Choosing identities in America.* Los Angeles, California: University of California Press.

Xie, Y. & Greenman, E. (2005). Segmented Assimilation Theory: A reformulation and empirical test. http://www.pse.isc.umich.edu/pubs/pdf/rr05-581.pdf. Downloaded July 14, 2007.

Zhou, M. & Xiong, G. S. (2005). The multifaceted American experiences of the children of Asian immigrants: Lessons for segmented assimilation. *Ethnic and Racial Studies, 28*(6), 1199-1152.

REFLECTIONS ON MULTICULTURALISM, ETHNIC-SENSITIVE PRACTICE, AND CULTURAL COMPETENCE

Multicultural Mistake

Charles Guzzetta

INTRODUCTION

The multiculturalism of the United States is a legitimate source of national pride, but the American society is not the first in which diversity of cultures was a major characteristic. Far from it. The history of societies around the entire world is replete with multicultural societies both small and vast. In fact, there has seldom been a significant period of time without a multicultural society since the earliest civilizations appeared.

MULTICULTURAL SOCIETIES THROUGHOUT HISTORY

The Roman Empire for hundreds of years united countless diverse cultures, traditions, religions, and societies, stretching all the way around the Mediterranean Sea and far inland. It was succeeded by the Moslem empire that grew swiftly in the seventh century and ultimately extended throughout the Middle East and North Africa, reaching deep into the Iberian Peninsula all the way to the Pyrenees in the west and to the gates of Vienna in the east. It was not expelled from Europe until the 20th century. In the 13th century, the Mongols had established the most extensive contiguous land empire the world has ever seen, incorporating innumerable cultures from the Yellow Sea to Poland. And then, in the 19th century, the British could legitimately boast that the sun never set on their empire, which included almost too many cultures to be counted, on every inhabited continent.

Multiculturalism is not a unique characteristic or contribution of the United States; it has seldom been absent from the world. What distinguishes multicultural America from all the others is that it was created by a process and presently exists in a form that can be found in none of its many antecedents. Multiculturalism is not new; it is American multiculturalism which is entirely new.

Of the many unique qualities that distinguish American multicultural society from all the many others, two are especially significant. The first relates to how past and most present multicultural societies have been created; the second relates to how those societies have been organized socially and politically.

Every major multicultural society, before the United States became the dominant global power, was created as a result of conquest. The Romans, the Moslems, the Mongols, the British and all the rest were aggressive, expansive, relentless empire-builders who became multicultural primarily because in their expansion, they swept over the many cultures in their paths and subjugated those cultures to the requirements of the triumphant empire. The subject cultures did not seek to enter the empires that overwhelmed them–any more than a fisherman seeks the storm that sweeps him into the sea. America, on the other hand, became multicultural by allowing successive waves of immigrants to cross its borders and to bring with them the cultures of their many homelands. The United States did not conquer and subjugate other cultures, with the regrettable exceptions of the Indians and the Mexicans of the Southwest.

Even with those exceptions, American's enchantment with imperialism was brief, and its pursuit of empire in the 19th century did not end when subject cultures broke free after prolonged and violent struggles, as happened to all other multicultural societies. The end of the American imperial period was signaled by the voluntary granting of independence to the Philippines in 1946 without those islands having had to fight for their freedom–and after less than 50 years of American occupation. It was an act virtually without precedent in the long annals of empire and was duplicated when the United States ceded the Canal Zone to Panama a few decades later.

From time to time, activist Puerto Ricans claim that their independence was taken by the United States, but this charge is absurd on its face. After the 16th century age of European exploration, Puerto Rico was never independent; in fact, it was freed by the United States from its exploited status as a minor colony of Spain. The aspirations to nationhood of some Puerto Ricans represent a demand for a presumed past status that the island never enjoyed; moreover, current island inhabitants themselves repeatedly have been given the opportunity to vote on their future status, including independence, and, in each election, they have chosen to remain within the United States as a commonwealth. These votes themselves have been remarkable. Perhaps no other country ever allowed one of its territories to vote for its independence–and then to have them freely reject it. Such is not the stuff of empires.

The other characteristic–social and political organization–of other multicultural societies differed significantly overall and in many specific ways from the situation in which diverse cultures exist within the United States. One key difference relates to the access provided for full and free participation in the governmental processes of the dominant culture. Even today, it is remarkably easy to become an American citizen and thereby to enjoy "all the rights and privileges thereunto appertaining." Not so in preceding multicultural societies.

Roman citizenship sometimes was granted to people from diverse cultures, but only under particular and limiting circumstances–and usually as a reward for exceptional service to the empire. Rights enjoyed by Roman citizens differed sharply from those exercised by people from the empire's other constituent cultures, with the result that Roman citizenship was very highly prized. The Book of Acts records one of the most famous examples of the privileges of Roman citizenship. When St. Paul's aggressive proselytizing of Jews became intolerable to the powerful priesthood, he was arrested and headed for a certain doom. Once he revealed that he was a Roman citizen, all attempts to prosecute him stopped at once; a Roman citizen could demand to be tried in Rome.

Moslems did not extend equal rights to the diverse people within their empire even after the occupied peoples converted to Islam. Converts attained a special status in Moslem society and were granted certain privileges that placed them above "infidels," but they remained below their Moslem masters. It was a kind of second-class citizenship which was an improvement over their former status, but well short of equality.

If you had not been born a Mongol, there was no possibility that you could expect ever to achieve equality in the Mongol empire. Mongols were tolerant of the diverse traditions and cultures of the peoples in the vast territory they conquered, but their tolerance was never considered equality. The long peace of the Mongols was not the peace of a democracy; it was the peace of a concentration camp. Few people in the diverse cultures within the Mongol empire ever had cause to misunderstand the difference between being a Mongol and not being a Mongol.

As recently as the 20th century, even while the great British Empire was disintegrating, its rulers made painfully clear that there was a significant difference between being born British and being a British subject. British subjects from commonwealth countries which had gained their freedom in Africa and Asia were putative British citizens, but when seeking to escape the upheavals in their newly-independent nations, they found themselves barred from entering England.

AMERICAN MULTICULTURALISM

In the United States, the situation is different from all these examples. Once a person attains U.S. citizenship, his rights as a citizen are the same as those of someone whose family has been in the country for generations. A naturalized citizen is simply a citizen, the same as every other citizen. Moreover, the path to American citizenship is not especially demanding. Merely being born in the country confers full citizenship, irrespective of the citizenship of the one's parents; to become naturalized citizens, aspirants who pass very modest requirements can achieve the status of full citizenship. Many Americans are not aware of how very unusual this policy is. For example, Germany still operates under the principle of *jus sanguinis*, which limits citizenship to those who can prove they have "German Blood." (Although in 2000, the law was changed to open the possibility that children born in Germany to immigrant parents might become eligible for citizenship.) Japan makes citizenship requirements so severe that few of the hundreds of thousands of immigrants from throughout Asia can hope ever to become Japanese citizens. In some Arab countries, those who hold citizenship represent a tiny minority of the population; the rest are not and never can become eligible for citizenship. The list goes on and on.

Many past societies that were intensely multicultural practiced admirable tolerance toward the various indigenous subcultures that were not appropriated by the ruling group. However, the notion that any or all of those many cultures were equal to the dominant culture, or ever could be equal, was simply never a serious consideration. Only in the United States is there the insistence and demand for an official government policy that holds all cultures to be entitled to equal recognition, acceptance and respect. Only in the United States may innumerable minor sects call themselves "cultures" and demand universal deference, even when they actively reject the principles and traditions of the dominant American culture.

The late historian Arthur Schlesinger, Jr. wrote that the "American culture" does not consist of being a White Protestant, but that it means acceptance of the fundamental principles of democracy. One concept of what comprises the elusive American "core culture" was expounded by Samuel P. Huntington; he included the English language, rule of law, freedom, representative government (implying restrictions on power of the government), equality, and the traditions of moral values and a work ethic. It is this core culture, he claimed, that makes an American an American.

The idea that American society in multicultural merely because it consists of many different cultures living within the borders of the country is at best naïve. Such an arrangement need not denote a real society at all. Under the dictatorship of Tito, the many diverse and antagonistic Balkan states were kept from engaging in their centuries-old attempts to annihilate each other. The fact that they never formed a true multicultural society was clear as soon as Tito died, and the country he had cobbled together broke into hostile states that immediately resumed their ancient blood feuds. There was no central society or set of social norms to which component states actually committed themselves. The inhabitants of Yugoslavia did not see themselves as Yugoslavians, but as they had seen themselves before: Serbs, Slavs, Croats and so on. They did not comprise a true multicultural society. A multicultural society is one in which there may be many different cultures which preserve elements of their unique traditions, but which come to hold these as subordinate to the dominant culture. To celebrate the diverse cultures in the United States primarily for their separateness is to invite disunity, disloyalty, and, ultimately, the possible dissolution of the Union itself.

The genius of the American republic has been its ability to absorb huge numbers of people from altogether different and sometimes antagonistic cultures and to let them retain a cultural identity which they brought with them, but always to do so within their transformation into Americans. An immigrant whose primary loyalty and identity remains fixed to the country and culture from which s/he came is neither a good member of that culture nor a good American. The central task of an immigrant to the United States is to become an American by renouncing foreign allegiances, but without having to renounce his/her foreign roots. This is not so daunting a task. Immigrants have been doing it, gladly, since before the country became a free nation. In fact, only in recent years has there been a serious attempt to shift the celebration of citizenship from the immigrant joy at becoming an American to celebrating the determination to remain something else while nevertheless enjoying the blessings of American citizenship.

The ability to keep faith with one's native culture while transferring one's principal commitment to the American core culture is the bedrock of our multiculturalism. Such a stance does not require losing one's former cultural identity nor seeking to be totally absorbed into the newly adopted culture; it simply means that one desires to be fully American, even if that often includes the popular and obtuse designation of hyphenating one's Americanism. The quintessential example of successful negotiation in the task of being both faithful to one's original culture and also completely loyal to a new, adopted culture is found in the long history of the Jews.

Perhaps nowhere is this more clearly and succinctly described than in *Jean Christophe*, the 1910 French masterpiece by Romain Rolland. He wrote:

> The Jews are quite erroneously reproached with not belonging to any nation and with forming . . . a homogeneous people impervious to the influence of the different races with which they have pitched their tents. In reality there is no race which more easily takes on the impress of the country . . . The autochthonous citizens of any country

have very little right to reproach the Jews with a lack of . . . national feeling of which they themselves possess nothing at all . . . [Jews] assume the . . . customs of the other country in which they live . . . without losing . . . the quality of their race.

One could reasonably argue that German Jews have always been the most German of Germans, Italian Jews the most Italian of Italians and similarly, American Jews the most American of Americans; they have become thoroughly committed citizens of any country in which they live, but all the while still proudly cherishing their Jewish culture. The concept is important but not complicated: One is an American who happens to be a Jew; not a Jew who happens to be an American. American multiculturalism based on this simple concept would make one an American who happened to have German or Spanish or Chinese or whatever else roots, not an Italian or Brazilian or whatever who happened to also be an American. Yet, despite the model Jews have set for multiculturalism, the benefits and special concerns that many advocates of multiculturalism demand for people whom they say add "diversity" to American society never seem to include Jews among those who should be carefully cultivated with special access to jobs, scholarships, and other enticements. It would seem that radical multiculturalists reserve the special favors for those who take pride in purposely remaining outside the normal bounds of American society in what could be seen as a rejection of the society that nurtures them in ways that their native society never did. The utter folly of the current trend among some Americans to glorify separateness of the diverse cultures which comprise the United States lies partly in its potential destructiveness to the American culture–one which makes true multiculturalism even possible.

The many cultures in the United States today join a long line of different populations that have become part of the country. Many, perhaps most of them, were not welcomed initially. Their differences made them seem alien and threatening to many of the other cultures already here. But the overwhelming majority of people who came to this country wanted to be Americans, and those who stayed soon found that it was entirely possible for them to retain key aspects of the cultures they had left while becoming fully American. This was possible because their former cultures, which they might continue to appreciate, became secondary to their identity as Americans. In most cases, that is what they wanted. The ideas that they should not learn English, should not have to work hard at whatever jobs they were able to get, need not exercise their voting franchise, and in other ways not accept the core American values would have been unimaginable to them. Those who perceived this country as being irretrievably hostile and nothing like their dreams always had a readily available alternative; they could leave. In fact, about 30% of all immigrants to the United States have gone back to their home countries for various reasons, including their rejection of what they perceived to be American culture. If they were unwilling or unable to become fully American, return may well have been the wisest course of action for them. It certainly made more sense than to remain in the United States, enjoying its manifold benefits while always holding themselves outside its core culture.

The nature of immigration has changed during the past half-century. Many former immigrants actually faced the necessity of making their immigration a one-way trip; total commitment to their adopted country may have seemed unfortunate but unavoidable, given the cost of returning. Today, travel opportunities offer the convenience of return for extended visits to native lands, however distant, and have made it possible for people to live in the United States and enjoy all its protections and benefits without feeling the tug of becoming a committed American. This status is not a recipe for building a nation; it is not good either for the immigrants or for the United States. Americans who cultivate the belief that immigrants can and perhaps even should maintain a primary loyalty to another culture need to study the effects of such a perspective in historical context.

This sort of thinking is rare anywhere else in the world. It would take an extraordinary imagination to visualize an American living in Poland feeling justified in insisting that the public schools teach his children in English. Or an American accused of a crime while living in Cuba expecting to enjoy the constitutional legal protections he would take for granted at home. Or an American convicted of a crime while in Saudi Arabia seriously believing that he should be immune to cruel corporal punishments. Or an American living in Zimbabwe feeling safe while raising (even modest) public objections to governmental corruption. The examples are endless.

MULTICULTURAL MISTAKE

The irony of the position of many multicultural advocates in the United States can be seen in their insistent demand that Americans overseas should scrupulously respect and adhere to the cultures of the countries in which they are living or traveling. Otherwise, it is asserted, such travelers and residents are fairly considered to be "ugly Americans." But people from other countries, living in the United States, should be allowed to follow the dictates of their own cultures. In other words, the extreme multiculturalists insist that Americans living in other countries should expect to be held to the rules of behavior of those countries, but immigrants living in the United States should be exempt from following the rules of the core culture of this country. Apparently, consistency is no more a virtue in such thinking than is patriotism.

This brand of multiculturalism has been held to be a hallmark of modern liberalism, but has been described as rather a new form of bigotry. As Michaels recently put it: "Diversity has become the left's way of doing neoliberalism," by seeking to suppress opposing ideas through accusations of "racism," "jingoism," and so on.

Social work practice which emphasizes difference over enculturation is perniciously misguided. Social work practice which concentrates on helping people retain their allegiance to a foreign culture after coming to the United States does harm to the country and does even more harm to the people social workers purport to assist by delaying the ability of immigrants to make the adaptations necessary to become truly American.

The settlement houses of the late 19th century often are cited as models for current multicultural emphasis on retaining one's foreign identity. Such an argument misses the point of early settlement house work. Social workers in settlement houses sought to mitigate the isolation, rejection, and oppression suffered by waves of immigrants who entered the country after the 1870's. The most convenient and effective way to afford relief was to help those dispirited and lonesome immigrants appreciate their own cultures *as they struggled to become Americans.* That is, while the cultures of the immigrants were being dismissed as inferior and offensive by some influential Americans, the settlement house workers helped segregated and depressed immigrants appreciate that the cultures they had left were worthy of preservation and respect even as the process of becoming American proceeded. It should be remembered that during that period of the country's history, some of the most bigoted assessments of immigrants issued from the highest places. The great liberal Theodore Roosevelt considered the "hordes" of recent immigrants inferior in every way; Woodrow Wilson refused to meet with them or their representatives. The situation of that time resembles in no way the present situation.

The objective of settlement house workers was not to help immigrants avoid committing to becoming Americans, but to help them gain the strength and self-respect to do so as rapidly and constructively as possible. Those early social workers understood what many social workers today do not seem to grasp: that immigrants grow more effectively and constructively from strength than from weakness. The purpose of helping immigrants build "self-esteem," that tiresomely overworked and misused concept, was to make them able more quickly and efficiently to adapt their lives and beliefs to the core culture of their adopted country, not to resist the process and to preserve their cultural differences. Jane Addams herself wrote of the hope that "inhabitants of this great nation might at last be united in a vast common endeavor for social ends." Unity was the ultimate objective of those social workers, not preservation of separateness. They understood the wisdom of their nation's motto: *E pluribus unum.*

Multiculturalism is one of the crowning glories of the United States. It demonstrates the country's success of bringing many different cultures together into a major culture of freedom and individuality; and to do so in collaboration with each other and with descendents of preceding immigrants' cultures. It is an idea based on mutuality rather than on suppression or preoccupation with alleged victimhood. It works because the denizens of the many different cultures who come to this country may retain key aspects of their identities while shifting their central loyalty to the core culture of their adoptive country. It promotes unity, not separatism, and views people from different cultures as enriching the country, not as Stoesz described the view of many current multiculturalists, as "aggrieved groups" who are seen as "victims of patriarchal, neocolonial politics."

If people from many different cultures continued indefinitely to retain their loyalty to their native cultures, they would not be able to create a single nation, but would comprise a multitude of mutually suspicious, competing sub-societies, until some superior power forced them all to submit, just as happened countless times in other societies that became multicultural. Social workers whose major aim is the protection of diverse cultures on an equal basis within the United States would do well to remember that such a state did once exist in the Western Hemisphere. Before Europeans came to the New World, it was populated by two major types of civilizations; those that were centrally organized and those that consisted of many different, separate, scattered cultures. The Aztec and Inca empires were rich, sophisticated, and accomplished multicultural societies which ruthlessly dominated the many unique cultures that existed within their respective empires. The Aztecs held bloody ritual sacrifices of its subject peoples–sometimes thousands in one ceremony– that were so brutal that they shocked even the Spanish conquistadors, who were no strangers to savagery. In fact, the few hundred Spanish soldiers who defeated the thousands of fierce warriors in the Aztec and Inca Empires owed their success to the assistance of innumerable subject peoples who greeted the Spanish as liberators, only to fall under another, almost equally brutal empire.

Conversely, before it was colonized, North American was populated by scores of separate Indian cultures, all fiercely protective of their own languages, customs, and unique identities, with the exception of the remarkable Iroquois Seven Nations. The marauding European settlers picked off each of the innumerable different Indian cultures in its turn until the entire continent had been swept clear of any significant Indian influence. Some Indian tribes survived and managed to preserve vestiges of their individual cultures by enduring banishment to barren reservations, dominated by the infamous Bureau of Indian Affairs, where success in remaining separate from the American mainstream culture has mainly produced, for the reservation Indians, squalid living conditions, rampant crime and alcoholism, and whatever satisfaction they may take from having stayed aloof from the dominant culture around them.

Those social workers who demand separateness and equal respect and status for every component culture in the United States are no friends of the people in those cultures and no friends of a united United States of America. One can picture how they would have debated in the 1850's, insisting that the unique Southern slave culture must be respected and accepted even if that meant the end of the Union. The efforts of some present-day social workers who agitate for separateness forestall or may even eliminate the day when the peoples of many cultures can become a true part of the fabric of this great nation.

Some multiculturalists are fond of referring to their image of the country as a great "mosaic." The image is wrong. If their position succeeded, what they would create is not a mosaic, but many scattered piles of rock. It is not each individual piece that is important in a mosaic; it is the final, overall picture created when the many different pieces are put together into one beautiful work of art. True, each colored bit of stone retains elements of its uniqueness, but alone, each is little more than a colored bit of stone. Their meaning and their beauty derives from how each becomes part of the whole, retaining its distinctive hue which it lends to the beauty of the completed mural. Social work's forever-active, ever-preaching multiculturalists may mean well, but their message is one of national fragmentation, not national unity. In these most perilous times for their country, their reckless message cannot be allowed to determine the course of their profession or of these United States.

REFERENCES

Addams, J. (1922). Peace and bread in time of war. New York: Women's International League for Peace and Freedom.

Huntington, S. (1996). The clash of civilizations and the remaking of world order. New York: Simon and Shuster.

Michaels, W. (2006). The trouble with diversity. *The American Prospect*, 17 (9) (September), 19-22.

Rolland, R. (1910). *Jean Christophe*. New York: Modern Library Edition.

Schlesinger, A. (1992). *The disuniting of America*. New York: Norton.

Stoesz, D. (2005). *Quixote's ghost*. New York: Oxford University Press.

Ethnic-Sensitive Practice: Contradictions and Recommendations

Alfreda P. Iglehart
Rosina M. Becerra

INTRODUCTION

The following discussion illuminates some of the contradictions and challenges that face the profession today as it attempts to provide ethnic-sensitive services. Contradictions can denote opposition, denial, inconsistency, and incongruity (*Merriam-Webster's Collegiate Dictionary*, 2005). Some are of a historical nature while others are in the realm of theoretical underpinnings, attitudes, and behaviors. The identification of these issues is a necessary first step in the problem-solving process.

This discussion is not about finger-pointing but, rather, about identifying issues so that fingers can be pointed in the appropriate direction for resolution. For this reason, each contradiction is followed by a recommendation for addressing it.

Background

It has been argued that unprecedented demographic changes coupled with greater visibility of racial/ethnic differences contribute to a need for competent practitioners who are skilled in working with diverse clients (Dhooper & Moore, 2001; Fong, 2004; Lum, 2003; Pumariega et al., 2005). The transformation of the American population is certainly indisputable. The United States Census Bureau (2006) noted that about one in every three United States residents is a member of a non-White group. Furthermore, the Census Bureau (2007), in a press release that reflects the news-worthiness of the information, announced that the minority population in the United States had surpassed 100 million. Hispanic residents are the largest minority group (44.3 million), followed by African Americans (40.2 million); Asians (14.9 million); American Indian and Alaska Natives (4.5 million); and Native Hawaiian and other Pacific Islanders (one million). Non-Hispanic White residents number about 199 million of the total population.

This ethnic/racial diversity appears to have the potential of altering the way social workers learn and practice their profession. This alteration is due, in part, to society and the profession's heightened awareness of the multitude of ways in which race/ethnicity affect intergroup attitudes, behaviors, and communication.

Although the merits and virtues of a multicultural and ethnic-sensitive education are widely debated, many in the field of social work apparently endorse education as a necessary intervention (Swank et al., 2001). This endorsement is visible in the growing body of literature on the development of models for teaching ethnic-sensitive social work practice (Swank et al., 2001). Examples of this growing body of work include Bankhead and Erlich (2005), Cox and Ephross (1998), Dhooper and Moore (2001), Hyde (1998), Jacobs and Bowles (1998), Lowery (2002), and Williams (2005).

Because the number of ethnic/racial minority groups in American society is too large for any worker to be knowledgeable about all of them (Cox & Ephross, 1998), emergent educational models often espouse a framework that is designed to be applicable across groups (Abrams & Gibson, 2007; Adams & Schlesinger, 1998; Devore, 2001; Lee & Greene, 2003). According to Lee and Greene (2003), some publications do target specific groups and provide instruction and research for social work practice with them. Work by Dhooper and Moore (2006), Fong (2004), and Stutters and Ligon (2001) would fall into this category.

Definition of Terms Used

A number of varying terms are used to capture social work with diverse populations. For example, "diversity practice" is broad enough to include groups defined by race/ethnicity, religious identification, sexual orientation, physical ability, social class, or age. "Multicultural practice" and "cultural competence" denote practice that is sensitive to the values, norms, beliefs, attitudes, folkways, behavior styles, and traditions that unite a group of people (Pinderhughes, 1989) and can also include race, ethnicity, gender, sexual orientation, and other aspects of a group's experiences that influence its worldview (Lum, 2003). Workers may engage in diversity practice and multicultural practice with White clients and communities that have traits and characteristics that define them as diverse and multicultural.

This article uses the term "ethnic-sensitive practice" to capture practice with, or on behalf of, ethnic/racial minority individuals and groups. "Ethnicity" encompasses social and psychological identity, values, norms, culture (language, food, dress, art, music) religion, and nationality (Cox & Ephross, 1998; Pinderhughes, 1989). "Race" denotes the biological and physical characteristics that separate one group from another and can have an ethnic dimension if group members have a defined way of life (Pinderhughes, 1989). "Minority" is used here to refer to nonWhite groups that differ in characteristics from the larger society and are subjected to differential treatment (*Merriam-Webster's Collegiate Dictionary*, 2005). Thus, Hispanics represent an ethnic minority group while African Americans, American Indians, Asians, Southeast Asians, and Pacific Islanders are racial minority groups. All are recognized as minority groups (Kim, 2003). This clarification is necessary because a number of terms are frequently used that may or may not have the same meaning. Ethnic-sensitive practice places the spotlight front and center on the ethnic and racial minority status of the client and client groups. Also, "minorities" will be used to mean ethnic and racial minority groups.

This background serves as the framework for considering the contradictions surrounding ethnic-sensitive practice and the framework for positing potential resolutions.

CONTRADICTIONS IN ETHNIC-SENSITIVE PRACTICE

While an emphasis on ethnic-sensitive practice is a testament to the profession's commitment to the provision of relevant, responsive services, a focus on teaching practitioners how to become more racially and ethnically sensitive only partially addresses issues in service delivery to ethnic/racial minorities. In the quest for relevant and effective service delivery, current identified approaches often mask a host of complexities and conundrums that accompany inter-ethnic/racial interactions.

Contradiction #1: Society Has Always Been Diverse

While the attention on ethnic-sensitive practice may be in response to the changing American racial/ethnic landscape, it is worth noting that American society has always been diverse. Diversity may not have historically existed the way it does currently, but the very origins of the social work profession are tied to the massive immigration of White ethnics to America–White ethnics who did not conform to the image of the "real" American. Iglehart and Becerra (1995) describe at length the role of this massive immigration in the development of the social work profession. These authors also provide an overview of the circumstances of other ethnic and racial groups in America during and after the Progressive Era and the nascent profession's response to them.

A major difference between then and now is not the *existence* of diversity in society but, rather, the *responses* to this diversity. With the

White ethnics, there was a belief that, over time, they would become as-similated into American society to the degree that their ethnicity would no longer be visible, and they would transform into true Americans. This assimilation would, of course, take a generation or two, but the outcome was the expected to yield the American melting pot. Thus, the Americanization movement supported efforts to eradicate the evidence of ethnicity and ethnic culture among the White ethnics by exposing them to the American way of life.

For groups that defied melting into the pot because they wore their ethnicity or race on their faces and in their culture, the profession had a variety of responses (Iglehart & Becerra, 1995). These responses included everything from denial of the group's existence to segregation and outright discrimination. Minority groups located in the West and Southwest were literally outside of the new profession's reach–a reach that was primarily associated with the burgeoning urbanization of the East.

In a content analysis of the literature on social work with minorities, DeVore (2001) and McMahon and Allen-Meares (1992) came to the same conclusion: social work seemed to have little interest in minorities and, when minorities were mentioned, there was a failure to address their social context. Lum (2003) defines context as the essential elements of an individual and his/her environment. For ethnic/racial minority groups, the social context would include stressors and their sources–both internal and external to the individual. By ignoring or minimizing the social context, the profession was, therefore, ignoring and minimizing the structural, institutional, and social factors that shape the minority group experience.

For some, this could mean that social work as a profession was racist, because to disregard a minority group's social context is to deny the role of discrimination in shaping their life experiences. Discounting the social context may seem reasonable, however, if few or no interventions are directed at the structural and institutional causes of problems. After all, social work as a profession is dominated by an emphasis on individual-level interventions (Haynes & Mickelson, 2006; Iglehart & Becerra, 1995; Leiby, 1978; Jansson, 2008; Martin & Martin, 1995). What appears as racism may actually be the nature of the profession itself–emphasis on individual-level practice.

For others, a lack of attention to social context may be reflective of the color-blind approach to social problems and service interventions. Color blindness denotes a sameness across populations (Bankhead & Erlich, 2005; Donnelly et al., 2005) so that problem definitions and problem solutions are unaffected by the characteristics of the clients. This is the "one-size-fits-all" notion that similar intervention techniques can be utilized with an array of problems and an array of populations (Bankhead & Erlich, 2005). In the color blind world, social context would have little or no relevance.

Regardless of whether social work has historically been racist or color blind in its dealings with ethnic/racial minority groups, the result is still the same: the social context of minority group has been minimized or disregarded in the development of sound intervention strategies. This is the history of the profession. With the growth of minority populations, the profession is making strides to alter its responses to these groups.

Recommendation #1: The Profession Should Accept Its Past

The past is the past and no effort at rewriting will erase it. One needed step in making peace with this past is acknowledging and accepting that the profession has made some mistakes and miscalculations as it has evolved. If past attempts to work with diverse populations mean that the profession was less sympathetic and less empathic than previously thought, then this admission is a step toward recovery and healing. Situations and circumstances do change, and the profession is changing along with them. Cox and Ephross (1998) cogently note that social workers are not expected to be perfect. In actuality, neither they nor the profession can lay claim to perfection. Using today's sensibilities, however, to accept, understand, and interpret the past can fortify the profession against perpetuating the same mistakes. These sensibilities should incorporate what Wright and Anderson (1998) identified as a need for the inclusion of clients' sociocultural and sociopolitical contexts in the service delivery process.

Instruction and training in ethnic-sensitive practice can be enhanced and more relevant when content on the profession's history is highlighted. With this content, learners gain an understanding of the profession's evolving efforts in service delivery to ethnic and racial minority groups. This knowledge base places workers in the context of the profession so that they know that the issues confronting them as individuals are also ones that have historically confronted the profession. Workers can then realize that, in becoming more ethnic-sensitive practitioners, they are growing as individual practitioners while also serving to advance the profession.

Contradiction #2: Ethnicity Is Still a Credential

The imparting of knowledge about ethnic-sensitive practice assumes that all practitioners can be taught to work with ethnic and racial minority individuals and communities. This assumption rings hollow in the face of historical and voluminous literature that touts the value of group members working with and taking care of their own. Evidence of this was recorded as far back as 1902 when the first African American woman was hired as a social worker with a New York Charity Organization Society. The COS secretary recognized the value of using African Americans for work among their own people, whose problems they could understand and whose needs they could well interpret (Jones, 1928).

Merton (1972) refers to an "insider doctrine" that polarizes society by boasts of each group having a claim to a monopoly of knowledge about itself. He noted that ascribed status was becoming a new credentialism. Variations on this theme abound and include the often quoted line, "You have to be one in order to understand one" (Merton, 1972, p. 15). This insider doctrine is so pervasive that examples are readily available. In one issue of the *Los Angeles Times* alone, two items appeared that capture the thrust of the doctrine. One item reported a lawsuit filed against Bank of America Corporation by five current and former minority employees alleging that the bank regularly assigned them to largely minority neighborhoods (*Los Angeles Times*, 2007). The other item was a letter to the editor penned by a California State Senator asserting that race matters in representative government. He also supported the efforts of African Americans to elect an African American to fill a vacant congressional seat in a district with 26 percent African American, 49 percent White, 19 percent Hispanic, and five percent Pacific Islander (Ridley-Thomas, 2007). The letter writer notes that voters tend to vote for candidates who are like them and share their concerns.

Ethnic/racial minority groups often form one group and White practitioners make up another group. As outsiders to the minority group, White social workers may have to work a great deal harder to prove that they are understanding, accepting, and unbiased. Even with the most diligent of effort, there may still be some hint of doubt and tension between the worker and client that may defy resolution.

The insider doctrine has been supported by empirical evidence. One such example is the research of Garcia and Van Soest (2000). In using vignettes to study faculty responses to critical classroom incidents about race, they found that ethnic minority professors selected answers that had higher responsiveness levels than did other groups. These researchers suggest that discriminatory experiences due to racial identity may be a factor in this outcome. In addition, they theorize that being exposed to oppression may enable individuals to empathize more and be more open to dealing with this topic. These findings could also lead to the conclusion that minority instructors are better able to impart knowledge about ethnic-sensitive practice than non-minority instructors.

Another example lies in the research on ingroup interactions. Kaiser (2003), in a qualitative study of a Hmong community, concluded that the context of culturally explicit communication patterns and the rules for communication contribute to the complexities of service delivery with this group. The rules and context may be difficult for an outsider to comprehend. Weathers et al. (2002) found that race influences the interpretation of emotional cues and members of minority groups are more accurate in their interpretations of other group members' meanings. This could mean that, in social work practice, the minority practitioner is a more accurate interpreter of facial expressions and verbal communication patterns of members of his/her group. The minority practitioner may also be skilled in deciphering ingroup dialogue that is laced with subtext and hidden meanings.

The assumption that minority groups would rather take care of their own is still held by some practitioners. For example, Donnelly et al. (2005), in a study of battered women's shelters in several Southern states, found that respondents thought that women of color preferred to handle problems in their own communities and did not always need services from mainstream (White) agencies.

When taken a degree further, the assumption that minority groups prefer to handle problems in their own communities may support the development of the ethnic agency (Iglehart & Becerra, 1995). Studies have indeed shown that ethnic/racial minority group members do better in ethnic agencies. This "do better" is captured in less premature termination and better client outcomes for these agencies (Hohman & Galt, 2001; Holley, 2003; Schrover & Vermeulen, 2005; Uba, 1982; Yeh et al., 1994; Zane, 1994). Holley (2003) suggests that outsiders can provide capacity building assistance and serve as advocates rather than provide direct service.

Theoretical literature also gives credence to the insider doctrine. Social identity theory (SIT) has been widely used throughout the discipline of psychology and adopted by popular culture (Brown, 2000; Hogg, 2006). It provides some fairly quick and easy explanations for why individuals appear to prefer to interact with and be around members of their own groups. With SIT, group identification, ingroup bias, intergroup discrimination, self-esteem, and stereotyping can be explained through group membership that gives rise to social identity. SIT distinguishes between personal and social identity with an emphasis on the social identity. It helps to explain why members of the same group can be found clustering together in schools, religious organizations, communities, work-site lunchrooms, and other locations in which the individual is able to use her/his discretion is selecting those with whom to interact.

SIT applies to all groups, not just to minority ones. Green et al. (2005), in a study of 257 White social workers' attitudes about people of color, found that the majority of respondents had positive attitudes about diversity. As a matter of fact, their attitudes were more positive than those of the public. Although White social workers were supportive of workforce equality for people of color, many were hesitant to express a desire for more closeness with them. Indeed, 85 percent of the respondents indicated that most of their best friends were from their own racial group.

If individuals prefer members of their own groups, and if this is the "natural order" of social contact, then ethnic-sensitive social work practice may be paddling against an overpowering current. While ethnic-sensitive instruction and education are offered, they may be insufficient in countering the insider doctrine and social identity theory.

Recommendation #2: Ethnic Credential Should Be Discussed

The ethnicity credential may be the elephant in the room that no one acknowledges; yet, most people may harbor some degree of adherence to it. When White practitioners speak on topics of race and ethnicity, there may be the unspoken question, "Why *is s/he* talking about this? What makes *her/him* an expert?" To openly raise this question may provoke reactions of defensiveness or even anger. In this climate of diversity, however, practitioners must not shy away from asking the difficult questions or raising the difficult issues. Giving voice to widely held thoughts may be a necessary first step to understanding the complexities of intergroup behavior.

Practitioners need to explore the circumstances that benefit from ethnic matching and those that do not. Not all clients want a worker who looks like them, and not all workers want a client who looks like them. The desired state of affairs could be one that allows for the exercise of choice. Perhaps a reasonable goal is for agencies to be able to meet the preferences of clients *and* workers regardless of what that preference may be. If this is the case, then the meaning and contribution of the ethnic credential to service delivery should be fully understood. Through acknowledging and accepting human behavior and all of its underpinnings, there is a greater openness to exploring the ethnic credential and its place, if any, in social work.

Contradiction #3: All Minority Groups Are Not the Same

The development of models for teaching ethnic-sensitive practice seems to imply that there is a similarity across all minority groups. The "sameness" approach emphasizes the commonalities across groups. This perspective may be necessary since the actual number of groups would exceed a worker's capacity to become expert in all of them. Dhopper and Moore (2001), for example, assert that many of these groups may differ from mainstream Americans in the following areas: meaning of family; place of religion; experience as Americans; poverty and lower economic status; level of acculturation; and culture-related disorders.

Teaching models highlight the knowledge and skills crucial for work with minorities. The knowledge is used to promote and support understanding in such areas as self, culture, cultural diversity, empowerment, ecological perspective, racism, power, prejudice, and oppression (Bankhead & Erlich, 2005; Cox & Ephross, 1998; Furuto, 2004; Lee & Greene, 2003; Lum, 2003b; Pinderhughes, 1989). The skills that are linked to ethnic-sensitive practice can include: communication and interviewing skills; assessment skills; process skills; conceptualization skills; mobilizing skills; and skills in participatory and evaluative research (Bankhead & Erlich, 2005; Cox & Ephross, 1998; Dhooper & Moore, 2001; Lum & Lu, 2003; Pinderhughes, 1989).

This knowledge development and skill acquisition do not broach the topic of status differential found among minority groups. While these groups may share the designation of "minority," they do not share the same status in American society. Each group has its own unique history, social context, and interface with White America. For example, Asian Americans are often considered the model minority–well-adjusted and with few psychological problems (Chen et al., 2003). This stereotype holds that they excel academically, are economically secure, and defeat barriers with family support and a strong work ethic (Cunanan et al., 2006). Thus, they may be victims of the benign neglect of the profession because of assumptions that they do not need social work assistance and that they take care of their own. While benign neglect is itself a form of discrimination, it is quite different from the discrimination faced by other minority groups.

Iglehart and Becerra (1995) detail the unique histories of America's minority groups. The social context, history, strengths, and needs of each group can differ markedly. Hispanic Americans have a history that is shaped by issues of immigration status that sharply divides the group into native born and foreign born. Native Americans' history is etched in efforts to eradicate an entire people. African Americans struggle to overcome a past marked by slavery, Jim Crow laws, and other overt acts of discrimination.

Models of teaching ethnic sensitive practice fail to take into account that some minorities are preferred over others in America. Dixon (2006), in a study that utilized survey and census data, revealed that the presence of large numbers of African Americans living near White respondents heightened their prejudice. African Americans represented a threat that raised levels of fear and hostility among this White population. The researcher also found that large numbers of Hispanics or Asians did not elicit the same response among the White respondents. As a matter of fact, White respondents who knew Hispanics and Asians were less prejudiced against them. This did not hold true for African Americans. Propinquity bred harmony for Hispanics and Asians, but hostility for African Americans.

African Americans appear to stand out among minority groups. The reasons for this may be tied to their history of slavery, discrimination, political mobilization, and continuous low rates on quality of life indicators. According to the U.S. Census Bureau (2007), California has 21 percent of the nation's minority population–the largest percent of any state. In comparison to Asians and Hispanics, African Americans in this state have higher poverty rates, unemployment rates, death rates in general, and infant death rates in particular (California Legislative Black Caucus, 2007). They also have lower home ownership rates and a lower household median income. On a national level, the African American population is also more segregated from non-Hispanic White population than are other minority groups (Iceland & Wilkes, 2006).

Many African Americans may think that terms such as "diversity" and "multiculturalism" shift attention from their needs to those of other groups. They may feel that their issues should have priority over those of other groups (Iglehart & Becerra, 1995). Surveys have found that many African American respondents believed that: (a) they are entitled to reparation from the government; (b) the democratic process should be altered in a manner that favors more responsiveness to their needs;

(c) they still suffer as a result of slavery and Jim Crow laws; (d) social class does not protect them from personal discrimination; and (e) the federal government is responsible for addressing inequities in employment, education, and health care (Chong & Kim, 2006; McGary, 2003).

White Americans may also define African Americans as the premier minority group and expect ameliorative strategies to specifically target this group. As Brown noted (1997), some people define race in terms of issues between the White and African American populations. This position may be a response to this group's political advocacy, outspoken leaders, White America's greater knowledge of this group than of other minority groups, and greater visibility throughout American history.

Commonalities do exist across minority groups; however, the differences between groups and how they are perceived by White America may be other issues that are virtually ignored.

Recommendation #3: Differences Should Be Acknowledged

Between group differences are significant enough to affect each group's interface with the larger society. Another step toward understanding the complexities of intergroup contact involves recognizing that all minority groups do not share a common status. Open discussion of these variations is one step toward creating an environment that fosters frankness and sharing. These discussions should include the topic of intergroup tensions and ways of resolving them. The questions of what determines group entitlement and whether one group has priority over another cannot be swept aside to avoid conflict. These discussions may not lead to answers, but they should lead to a greater understanding of the issues.

Within group differences also require more attention. The use of broad categorizations such as Asian Americans and Hispanics masks the heterogeneity found within these categorizations. Numerous researchers advocate for the disaggregating of sweeping categories so that greater attention can be devoted to more specialized intervention (Castex, 1994; Kim, 2006; Kramer & Nash, 1995; Leong et al., 1995; Tran & Dhooper, 1996).

Contradiction #4: Self-Awareness Is Not the Key

In ethnic-sensitive social work practice, self-awareness reigns as the critical, essential, crucial, and necessary element (Dhooper & Moore, 2001; Lee & Greene, 2003; Pinderhughes, 1989). Social workers are assumed to need to explore, examine, question, and be aware of their own assumptions, attitudes, behaviors, and values in order to be receptive to and benefit from ethnic-sensitive learning. Much of the teaching and training used for ethnic-sensitive practice devotes significant time to self-awareness discussion and self-awareness exercises.

Self-awareness discussions and exercises, however, are deemed crucial for White practitioners who are blind to their whiteness and the status it affords them (Adams & Schlesinger, 1988; Pinderhughes, 1989). Apparently, as White individuals, they must learn about culture (their own and that of others), diversity, social injustice, and oppression in order to grow as ethnic-sensitive practitioners. Differential treatment and numerous other forms of racism and discrimination make minority group members keenly aware of their color, culture, and other characteristics. Although ethnic/racial awareness becomes firmly stamped on the psyche of minority groups, awareness of whiteness seems to be missing for many within the White population. This self-awareness seems to be needed for White social workers regardless of their area of practice. For example, according to Bankhead and Erlich (2005:64), White liberal community organizers have their own struggles, issues, and complexities that may diminish their effectiveness as social change agents with culturally different populations.

For White practitioners, self-awareness also means examining White privilege and its association with unearned advantage and domination (Lowery, 2002). According to Donnelly et al. (2005:6), White privilege refers to a system of benefits, advantages, and opportunities experienced by White persons in American society simply because of their skin color. Workers must, therefore, unlearn and undo those patterns associated with social privilege (Swigonski, 1996).

A focus on worker self-awareness and White privilege has often been met with resistance from White workers (Abrams & Gibson, 2007). This should not be surprising since many well-intentioned, well-educated workers are dismayed to be treated as if they were contributing to the "minority problem." Placing White workers under the self-awareness microscope seems to imply some deficiency on their part. For workers who take pride in their open and supportive ethnic/racial attitudes and behaviors, this can come as quite a shock. Many feel justified in questioning the utility of the concept of White privilege and may extend that questioning to the validity of the instruction. Ethnic-sensitive trainers must then attempt to help learners move beyond their anger and anxiety so that the next stages of White identity development can be addressed (Abrams & Gibson, 2007). The resistance is generally interpreted as discomfort that is necessary for growth, self-awareness, and transformation.

The unlearning of firmly entrenched attitudes and behaviors cannot take place in a classroom over a short period of time. It may take a long time for people to change beliefs they have had for most of their lives about their own and other people's race and ethnicity–even when they are inaccurate (Bourjolly et al., 2005). In writing of the changing landscape of adult learning theory, Merriam (2004) reveals that learning has moved beyond being just a cognitive process located in the mind. The learning process is shaped by cultural, social, economic, and political forces. This could mean that bringing social workers together in a classroom-like setting to teach ethnic-sensitive practice ignores their social context and the social context of the learning process.

Pointing the finger at the worker has another major limitation. Worker attitudes are but one factor in the service delivery equation. Social work practice takes place in an organizational, community, and societal context. A change in worker attitudes may not result in a change in organizational structures and processes. A change in worker attitudes may not result in a change in the quality of life of minority communities. A change in worker attitudes may not result in a change in discriminatory or benign social policies. Some of the problems in service delivery to minority clients and communities may be the result of organizational practices that limit access, resources, and services for minorities. According to Holloway and Brager (1977), worker attitudes and behaviors may be too easily blamed for organizational problems, structures, programs, or ideology. People change appears to take priority over change at other system levels.

Recommendation #4: An Expanded Focus Is Needed

Focus should be expanded to include interventions that support ethnic-sensitive practice at the agency level. If ethnic-sensitive practice is placed in a systems perspective or in an ecological perspective, it is clear that the worker shares center stage with other actors and elements. As the profession continues to illuminate the need for effective ethnic-sensitive practice, these other elements should be drawn into the light. For example, in order for workers to engage in ethnic-sensitive practice, they will need support, encouragement, and incentives from the agency. Incentives are particularly important, because worker behaviors that are desired by the agency should be rewarded. Worker evaluations have to assess the worker in areas of ethnic-sensitive practice and link rewards to effectiveness in these areas.

Examination of organizational structures and processes should be undertaken to uncover those that inhabit and impede ethnic-sensitive practice. Workers practice their profession in an organizational context and worker acquisition of new learning may be powerless in overcoming agency limitations. Agency recruitment and retention policies/practices, outreach strategies, and advocacy activities are key factors in ethnic-sensitive practice. Agencies have to assess their norms, behaviors, processes, culture, and modes of interacting with minority clients (Fong & Gibbs, 1995). Unfortunately, as Brown (1997, p. 225) noted, diversity training tends to conveniently avoid addressing the need for dramatic changes in most organizational cultures and power structures.

The commitment of agency leadership to ethnic-sensitive practice cannot be overlooked. Administrators must have leadership skills, vision, and commitment in order to move an agency closer to achieving the goals of ethnic-sensitive practice. In addition, ethnic-sensitive management of a diverse staff reaffirms the agency's commitment to ethnic-sensitive worker-client relations. Workers who feel disempowered, alienated, or marginalized may not be receptive to any new learning the agency has to offer.

Focus should also be expanded to include elements outside of the agency. It may be difficult for an agency to engage in ethnic-sensitive practice if its task environment and general environment challenge that practice. Hasenfeld (1983) discusses these environments and provides their definitions. The task environment is a set of organizations and groups with which the organization exchanges resources and services while the general environment is composed of resources, population, technology, and culture. Because agencies are dependent on their environments (Hasenfeld, 1983; Schmid, 2004), practices occurring in the agency are influenced by the environment outside the agency. It may be virtually impossible for workers to offer ethnic-sensitive services if the task and general environments: (a) question this practice; (b) do not have positive regard for specific minority groups; (c) do not provide the necessary resources to support this practice; (d) and contain social policies that constrain and restrict worker efforts. As a consequence, advocacy at the community and policy levels becomes a crucial skill (Haynes & Mickelson, 2006).

When worker training is mandated, focus should expand to more fully include the training needs of minority workers when they are present in the agency. The assumption that the White worker is the only worker who needs ethnic-sensitive training ignores minority workers. Within and between group differences suggest that minority workers also have their own attitudes and behaviors that can benefit from examination and exploration. Each group has its own biases toward other groups and toward its own subgroups. Minority group status does not render one immune to ethnic/racial bias. The profession should foster a more inclusive ideology toward ethnic-sensitive practice.

When White workers are the intended beneficiaries of ethnic-sensitive training, perhaps the focus should not include the concept of White privilege. The resistance of White workers to this concept may have some legitimacy. It may be viewed as an indictment against them and create many more problems than solutions. It may not be essential for White workers to recognize, accept, or embrace this concept as they learn the tools and techniques of ethnic-sensitive practice. The introduction of this concept may erect a barrier that drains time, attention, and energy from the educational goals. Race and ethnic issues are controversial enough without the injecting of additional controversy. Trainers and educators should ask themselves, "Can ethnic-sensitive practice be taught without the concept of White privilege?"

CONCLUSION

The profession can no longer persist in approaching ethnic-sensitive practice as something that can be primarily taught at the worker level and still expect major change. The profession's social context dictates other interventions and other considerations. The United States has never been a race neutral society. Race and ethnicity pervade just about every aspect of society. In 1982, Hopps wrote that although many forms of exclusionary and discriminatory practices are numerous, "none is so deeply rooted, persistent, and intractable as that based on color" (Hopps, 1982, p. 3). Decades later, the intractability of race and ethnicity still exists. The issue of race and ethnicity is laden with emotion and surrounded by sensitivity. For these reasons, ethnic-sensitive practice cannot be taught the way other social work topics are taught.

The profession is altering its response to ethnic/racial diversity and that response should tackle an examination of the place of the ethnic credential in ethnic-sensitive practice, the differential status of minority groups, the over-reliance on self-awareness, and the need for intervention at other levels in the service delivery process. Ethnic-sensitive practice calls for open, frank discussions of between group and within group issues, issues that can be quite controversial. It calls for both micro and macro interventions–interventions that pertain to workers, administrators, agencies, the larger community, and social policies. In its journey toward more effective ethnic-sensitive practice, pathways should entail the fostering of climates that support meaningful training/education, meaningful agency change, and meaningful community and policy advocacy.

REFERENCES

Abrams, L. S., & Gibson, P. (2007). Reframing multicultural education: Teaching white privilege in the social work curriculum. *Journal of Social Work Education*, 43(1), 147-160.

Adams, A., & Schlesinger, S. (1988). Group approach to training ethnic sensitive practitioners. In C. Jacobs & D. Bowles (Eds.). *Ethnicity and race: Critical concepts in social work*. Silver Spring, MD: NASW Press.

Bankhead, T., & Erlich, J. (2005). Diverse populations and community practice. In M. Weil (Ed.). *The handbook of community practice*. Thousand Oaks, CA: Sage.

Bourjolly, J. N., Sands, R. G., Solomon, P., Stanhope, V., Pernell-Arnold, A., & Finley, L. (2005). The journey toward intercultural sensitivity: A non-linear process. *Journal of Ethnic & Cultural Diversity in Social Work*, 14, 41-62.

Brown, C. D. (1997). An essay: Diversity and unspoken conflicts. In C. D. Brown, C. C. Snedeker, & B. Sykes (Eds.). *Conflict and Diversity*. Cresskill, NJ: Hampton Press.

Brown, R. (2000). Social identity theory: Past achievements, current problems and future challenges. *European Journal of Social Psychology*, 30, 745-778.

California Legislative Black Caucus. (2007). *The state of Black California*. Sacramento: Author. http://democrats.assembly.ca.gov/members/a47/Stateblack.htm, Retrieved 5-29-07.

Carr-Ruffino, N. (1996). *Managing diversity: People skills for a multicultural workforce*. Cincinnati, OH: Thomson Executive Press.

Castex, G. M. (1994). Providing services to Hispanic/Latino populations: Profiles in diversity. *Social Work*, 39, 288-296.

Chen, S., Sullivan, N. Y., Lu, Y., & Shibusawa, T. (2003). Asian Americans and mental health services: A study of utilization patterns in the 1990s. *Journal of Ethnic & Cultural Diversity in Social Work*, 12, 19-42.

Chong, D., & Kim, D. (2006). The experience and effects of economic status among racial and ethnic minorities. *American Political Science Review*, 100, 335-351.

Cox, C. B., & Ephross, P. H. (1998). *Ethnicity and social work practice*. New York: Oxford University Press.

Cunanan, V. L., Guerrero, A. P. S., & Minamoto, L. Y. (2006). Filipinos and the myth of model minority in Hawai'i. *Journal of Ethnic & Cultural Diversity in Social Work*, 15, 167-192.

Devore, W. (2001). Ethnic sensitivity: A theoretical framework for social work practice. In L. Dominelli, W. Lotenz, & H. Soydan (Eds.). *Beyond racial divides: Ethnicities in social work practice*. Burlington, VT: Ashgate Publishing.

Dhooper, S. S., & Moore, S. E. (2001). *Social work practice with culturally diverse people*. Thousand Oaks, CA: Sage.

Dixon, J. C. (2006). The ties that bind and those that don't: Toward reconciling group threat and contact theories of prejudice. *Social Forces*, 84, 2179-2204.

Donnelly, D. A., Cook, K. J., Ausdale, D. V., & Foley, L. (2005). White privilege, color blindness, and services to battered women. *Violence Against Women*, 11, 6-37.

Fong, L. G., & Gibbs, J. T. (1995). Facilitating services to multicultural communities in a dominant culture setting: An organizational perspective. *Administration in Social Work*, 19, 1-24.

Fong, R. (2003). Cultural competence with Asian Americans. In D. Lum (Ed.). *Culturally competent practice*. Pacific Grove, CA: Thomson-Brooks/Cole.

Fong, R. (2004). Overview of immigrant and refugee children and families. In R. Fong (Ed.). *Culturally competent practice with immigrant and refugee children and families*. New York: Guilford Press.

Furuto, S. B. C. L. (2004). Theoretical perspectives for culturally competent practice with immigrant children and families. In R. Fong (Ed.). *Culturally competent practice with immigrant and refugee children and families*. New York: Guilford Press.

Garcia, B., & Van Soest, D. (2000). Facilitating learning on diversity: Challenges to the professor. *Journal of Ethnic & Cultural Diversity in Social Work*, 9, 21-39.

Green, R. G., Kiernan-Stern, M., & Baskind, F. R. (2005). White social workers' attitudes about people of color. *Journal of Ethnic & Cultural Diversity in Social Work*, 14, 47-68.

Hardina, D., Middleton, J., Montana, S., & Simpson, R. (2007). *An empowering approach to managing social service organizations*. New York: Springer.

Hasenfeld, Y. (1983). *Human service organizations*. Englewood Cliffs, NJ: Prentice-Hall.

Haynes, K. D., & Mickelson, J. S. (2006). *Affecting change–Social workers in the political arena*. Sixth Edition. New York: Pearson–Allyn and Bacon.

Hogg, M. A. (2006). Social identity theory. In P. J. Burke (Ed.). *Contemporary social psychological theories*. Stanford, CA: Stanford University Press.

Hohman, M. M., & Galt, D. H. (2001). Latinas in treatment: Comparisons of residents in a culturally specific recovery home with residents in a non-specific recovery home. *Journal of Ethnic & Cultural Diversity in Social Work*, 9, 93-109.

Holley, L. C. (2003). Emerging ethnic agencies: Building capacity to build community, *Journal of Community Practice*, 11, 39-57.

Holloway, S., & Brager, G. (1977). Some considerations in planning organizational change. *Administration in Social Work*, 1, 349-357.

Hopps, J. (1982). Oppression based on color. *Social Work*, 27, 3-5.

Hyde, C. (1998). A model for diversity training in human service agencies. *Administration in Social Work*, 22, 19-36.

Iceland, J., & Wilkes, R. (2006). Does socioeconomic status matter? Race, class, and residential segregation. *Social Problems*, 53, 248-273.

Iglehart, A. P., & Becerra, R. M. (1995). *Social services and the ethnic community*. Boston: Allyn and Bacon. Reissued–Prospect Heights, IL: Waveland Press, 2000.

Jacobs, C., & Bowles, D. (Eds.). (1998). *Ethnicity and race: Critical concepts in social work*. Silver Spring, MD: NASW Press.

Jansson, B. S. (2008). *Becoming an effective policy advocate.* Fifth Edition. Belmont, CA: Thomson brooks/Cole.

Jones, E. (1928). Social work among Negroes. *The Annals of the American Academy of Political and Social Science,* 240, 287-293.

Kaiser, T. L. (2003). Achieving shared meaning in cross-cultural dialogue: Understanding a Hmong family's response to marital violence. *Journal of Ethnic & Cultural Diversity in Social Work,* 12, 29-54.

Kim, W. (2006). Diversity among Southeast Asian ethnic groups: A study of mental health disorders among Cambodians, Laotians, Miens, and Vietnamese. *Journal of Ethnic & Cultural Diversity in Social Work,* 15, 83-100.

Kim, Y. S. E. (2003). Understanding Asian-American clients problems and possibilities for cross-cultural counseling with special reference to Korean Americans. *Journal of Ethnic & Cultural Diversity in Social Work,* 12, 91-114.

Kramer, K. D., & Nash, K. B. (1995). The unique social ecology of groups: Findings from groups for African Americans affected by sickle cell disease. *Social Work with Groups,* 18, 55-65.

Lee, M. Y., & Greene, G. J. (2003). A teaching framework for transformative multicultural social work education. *Journal of Ethnic & Cultural Diversity in Social Work,* 12, 1-28.

Leiby, J. (1978). *A history of social welfare and social work in the United States.* New York: Columbia University Press.

Leong, F. T., Wagner, N. S., & Tata, S. P. (1995). Racial and ethnic variations in help-seeking attitudes. In J. G. Ponterotto, J. M. Casas, L. A. Suzuki, & C. M. Alexander (Eds.). *Handbook of multicultural counseling.* Thousand Oaks, CA: Sage.

Los Angeles Times. (2007). BofA accused of racial bias. May 19.

Lowery, C. T. (2002). Diversity, ethnic competence, and social justice. In M. A. Mattaini, C. T. Lowery, & C. H. Meyer (Eds.). *Foundations of social work practice.* Third Edition. Washington, DC: NASW Press.

Lum, D. (2003a). Culturally competent practice. In D. Lum (Ed.). *Culturally competent practice.* Second Edition. Pacific Grove, CA: Thomson–Brooks/Cole.

Lum D. (2003b). Knowledge acquisition. In D. Lum (Ed.). *Culturally competent practice.* Second Edition. Pacific Grove, CA: Thomson–Brooks/Cole.

Lum, D. (2003c). Social context. In D. Lum (Ed.). *Culturally competent practice.* Second Edition. Pacific Grove, CA: Thomson–Brooks/Cole.

Lum, D., & Lu, Y. E. (2003). Skill Development. In D. Lum (Ed.). *Culturally competent practice.* Second Edition. Pacific Grove, CA: Thomson–Brooks/Cole.

Martin, E. P., & Martin, J. M. (1995). *Social work and the black experience.* Washington, DC: NASW Press.

McGary, H. (2003). Achieving democratic equality: Forgiveness, reconciliation, and reparations. *The Journal of Ethics,* 7, 93-113.

McMahon, A., & Allen-Meares, P. (1992). Is social work racist? A content analysis of recent literature. *Social Work,* 37, 533-539.

Merriam, S. B. (2004). The changing landscape of adult-learning theory. In J. Coming, B. Garner, & C. Smith (Eds.). *Review of adult learning and literacy*: Vol. 4: *Connecting research, policy, and practice.* Mahwah, NJ: Lawrence Erlbaum Associates Pubishers.

Merriam-Webster's Collegiate Dictionary. (2005). Eleventh Edition. Springfield, MA: Merriam-Webster Incorporated.

Merton, R. K. (1972). Insiders and outsiders: A chapter in the sociology of knowledge. *American Journal of Sociology,* 78, 9-47.

Pumariega, A. J., Rogers, K., & Rothe, E. (2005). Culturally competent systems of care for children's mental health: Advances and challenges. *Community Mental Health Journal,* 41, 539-555.

Ridley-Thomas, M. (2007). Letter to the editor. *Los Angeles Times,* May 19, 2007.

Rodriguez, J. (2006). Color-blind ideology and the cultural appropriation of hip-hop. *Journal of Contemporary Ethnography,* 35, 645-668.

Schmid, H. (2004). Organization-environment relationships: Theory for management practice in human service organizations. *Administration in Social Work,* 28, 97-113.

Schmidt, S. L. (2005). More than men in white sheets: Seven concepts critical to the teaching of racism as systematic inequality. *Equity and Excellence in Education,* 38, 110-122.

Schrover, M., & Vermeulen, F. (2005). Immigrant organizations. *Journal of Ethnic and Migration Studies,* 31, 823-832.

Strutters, A., & Ligon, J. (2001). Differences in refugee anxiety and depression: Comparing Vietnamese, Somalian, and former Yugoslavian clients. *Jouornal of Ethnic & Cultural Diversity in Social Work,* 10, 85-96.

Swank, E., Asada, H., & Lott, J. (2001). Student acceptance of a multicultural education: Exploring the role of a social work curriculum, demographics, and symbolic racism. *Journal of Ethnic & Cultural Diversity in Social Work,* 10, 85-103.

Swigonski, M. W. (1996). Challenging privilege through Afrocentric social work practice. *Social Work,* 41, 153-161.

Tran, T. V., & Dhooper, S. S. (1996). Ethnic and gender differences in perceived needs for social services among three elderly Hispanic groups. *Journal of Gerontological Social Work,* 25, 121-147.

Uba, L. (1982). Meeting the mental health needs of Asian Americans: Mainstream or segregated services. *Professional Psychology,* 13, 215-221.

U. S. Bureau of the Census. (2006). Nation's population one-third minority. Press release dated May 10. Washington, DC: Author. <http://www.census.gov/Press-Release> Retrieved May 18, 2007.

U. S. Bureau of the Census. (2007). Minority population tops 100 million. Press Release dated May 17, 2007. Washington, DC: Author. <http://www.census.gov/Press-Release> Retrieved May 18, 2007.

Weathers, M. D., Frank, E. M., & Spell, L. A. (2002). Differences in the communication of affect: Members of the same race versus members of a different race. *Journal of Black Psychology,* 28, 66-77.

Williams, C. C. (2005). Training for cultural competence: Individual and group processes. *Journal of Ethnic & Cultural Diversity in Social Work,* 14, 111-143.

Wright, O. L., Jr., & Anderson, J. P. (1998). Clinical social work practice with urban African American families. *Families in Society: The Journal of Contemporary Human Services,* 79, 197-214.

Yan, M. C., & Wong, Y. R. (2005). Rethinking self-awareness in cultural competence: Toward a dialogic self in cross-cultural social work. *Families in Society,* 86, 181-188.

Yeh, M., Takeuchi, D., & Sue, Stanley. (1995). Asian-American children in the mental health system: A comparison of parallel and mainstream outpatient service centers. *Journal of Clinical and Child Psychology, 23,* 5-12.

Zane, N., Hatanaka, H., Park, S., & Akutsu, P. (1994). Ethnic specific mental health services: Evaluation of the Parallel approach for Asian-American Clients. *Journal of Community Psychology, 22,* 68-81.

Lessons from Marrano Beach: Attachment and Culture

Rita Ledesma

INTRODUCTION

This essay offers reflections derived from practice and research that support the thesis that effective practice requires the development of capacities that support engagement across cultures. Difference and social, political, and cultural borders are always negotiated in every social work arena of practice. A strong theoretical perspective and a capacity for self-reflection can result in practice that situates individual, family, and community strengths and challenges within the context of broader human experience. The broad parameters of human experience include social, historical, ecological, and political context, culture, attachment experiences, and exposure to loss and trauma.

I have worked as a caseworker, clinician, administrator, and organizer. My career has addressed child and family focused issues within the urban Los Angeles community. Areas of expertise include practice within poor, Latino/a and American Indian/Alaska Native urban Los Angeles communities, but my experience has not been limited to these communities. In the last fifteen years, professional roles converged and shifted as I entered academia and took on the identity of practitioner-scholar. Throughout my academic career, I remained very close to community based practice by providing consultative services and clinical supervision at local child and family focused organizations.

There is a reciprocal relationship between practice, scholarship, and teaching. Practice informs my research agenda, and the findings from research influence practice and teaching. Teaching is designed to prepare students for cross-cultural practice in the local community. As I (temporarily) move away from the classroom to assume other positions in the University community, it seems an appropriate time to reflect on the things that I have learned and to consider the elements of practice and scholarship that I believe are helpful in meeting the needs of the local community. These elements include developing a strong theoretical foundation, cultural knowledge, and capacities for self-reflection. Each element is linked, because theoretical perspectives support examination and analysis of cultural material and human behavior, experiences, and events, and self-reflection promotes abilities to engage across cultures, to make appropriate use of self (including disclosures that meet client/constituent needs), and to establish boundaries and parameters in relationships. From clients (my best teachers), supervisors, consultants, students, and study, I have learned about the role of theory, the significance of culture, and the importance of reflection and consultation.

CAREER TRAJECTORY

In 1979, I entered a Masters in Social Welfare program. This decision to pursue a career in social work was influenced by Chicano/a social workers who integrated concerns about the local community, social justice, and attention to cultural material in professional practice. These social workers, and specifically, Margarita Mendez, served as role models and mentors who supported the development of a social work practice that is grounded in the local community, attentive to cultural material, individual and community strengths, socio-political context, and fiercely committed to social justice. After graduation, I worked in a variety of settings providing direct service as well as serving in leadership and administrative capacities. Client populations included children, adolescents, adults and families, veterans, victims of family and community violence, rape survivors, and college students. In 1989, I began a doctorate program in social welfare, and I continued work as a clinician in community organizations and in private practice. My research examined cultural influences on family development, loss, bereavement, and health. I began my teaching career as an adjunct faculty in 1992 and accepted a tenure track position in 1995. I taught practice and human behavior courses in the School of Social Work's undergraduate and graduate programs. Throughout my career, I actively engaged with organizations that advance a culturally focused agenda and that link this agenda to social justice concerns.

I currently direct a peer mentoring program for freshmen students at a large urban university, where the majority of students are first generation college students and Latino/a, and I am the president of the campus chapter of the California Faculty Association, a statewide labor union that represents faculty (tenure track and lecturers), counselors, librarians, and coaches. This discussion of career trajectory illustrates the scope of my social work practice and expertise. The comments in this essay reflect evaluation of this practice at the mid-point of my career and efforts to integrate micro and macro level interventions with a culturally focused and activist agenda that is theoretically sound and reflective and *useful* to constituents.

LESSONS LEARNED: THE ROLE OF THEORY

It is critical to develop a theoretical stance that serves as the foundation for practice at all levels. Analysis of individual behavior, community development or social policy requires the capacity to think conceptually and strategically about the cultural, social, political, and ecological context wherein the unit of analysis is situated. This approach supports capacities to investigate the etiology, process, and short/long-term consequences of the issue. From this perspective, it becomes possible to elicit an "emic/insider" perspective, to interpret the issue from the perspective of the actor, to examine how the issue is socially constructed, and to explore why/how the issue is sustained and the range of possible alternatives.

Social workers can develop a theoretical orientation that resonates with personal values, that is consistent with professional values and ethics, and that advances the work *from the perspective of the client, community or constituency.* The most elaborate and sophisticated theories are meaningless unless they actually prove useful to clients, communities, and constituents. I tend to link an activist and progressive social justice orientation to the analysis of individual, family, and community distress that situates the client in context, and this orientation influences how I evaluate the utility of theory. Does the theory advance my understanding and capacity to interpret and accurately reflect the human and social conditions in front of me? It also is critically important that theory allow me to make my skills and expertise available to clients/constituents. In practice, I integrate theory that helps me engage cross-culturally with clients, communities, and constituents and that helps me understand the influences of the broader cultural, social, political, and historical context on development and social problems. I am interested in developing intervention strategies (individual, family or group therapy; community organizing; programs; training, educational, and research activities) that support the interpretation of life events and facilitate transformational and liberation processes that the client/constituent evaluates as appropriate for individual life circumstance. A quote by Archbishop Oscar Romero, who was assassinated in El Salvador in 1980 as he was saying Mass, has greatly influenced my orientation, "Psychological problems caused by social conditions can not be solved by psychological means alone."

The theories that explain human development and human behavior that resonate most with this perspective include psychosocial theories of development, theories that advance understanding on the nature of attachment and loss, and theories that examine culture, strengths, and the stories of clients and communities. Psychosocial developmental theories are useful, because social workers need a language and structure for evaluating the degree to which the developmental tasks associated with productivity and well-being in this society are mastered. I often say to students that they need to be able to draw on this knowledge in the same way in which they breathe. Therefore, Eriksonian and life-span/ life-cycle perspectives have proved useful. It is important to integrate understanding about the resolution of developmental tasks in context, because access to services and interventions frequently are focused on the identification and management of pathology. The explanation for the condition often prescribes the intervention. If we are to avoid patholo- gizing behavior, developmental process must be interpreted to account for the complexity that so often characterizes the human condition.

It is critically important to understand the expansiveness and quality of the support network and the mechanisms that influence the development of personality. What is the nature and quality of attachment experiences with family, community, and culture? What resources are available to encourage and support development and engagement with the world? Attachment theory, relational perspectives, social constructivist and perspectives that explore loss and trauma have proven invaluable to my practice and scholarship. Theories that support the analysis of culture in the context of relationships of power and political-historical moment provide the foundation for much of my conceptual thinking about how development unfolds, how challenges are negotiated, and how strength and resilience manifest. These theoretical perspectives are integrated in practice by invoking strengths-based and narrative approaches in the design and evaluation of interventions.

These perspectives, specifically theories associated with Cultural Studies, have advanced capacities to expand and integrate knowledge about the influence of policy, and social and historical events on indi- vidual and community development. This has provided a structure for examining the consequences of policy and socio-political conditions on developmental processes, attachment experiences, and exposure to loss and trauma. Social justice concerns are implicated in this analysis, be- cause frequently, developmental processes and loss and traumatic expe- riences are the result of policy and socio-political conditions. I have written about this relationship with reference to the American Indian/ Alaska Native experience.

Another clear example of these phenomena is apparent in the post- Katrina activities in New Orleans. Although the hurricane was a natural event, the social policies and interventions provided in the aftermath may prove to have long term disastrous effects for individual, family, and community development. As a result of the losses associated with the event, attachments to family, community, and cultural touchstones have been severed, and the consequences will likely have intergenerational effects. Federal and local policy may exacerbate the losses and trauma that residents experience. Suppose that a family, who was displaced by Hurricane Katrina, presented for services at an agency in Los Angeles. The social worker's ability to engage, to attend to concerns, to gather relevant history, and to establish a relationship with the family is influenced by the worker's capacity to examine, interpret, and reflect concerns from a sound theoretical framework that includes attention to development, attachment, culture, and context.

The human behavior in the social environment courses which I developed and teach at the CSULA School of Social Work are designed to promote understanding of the issues discussed in this section. The sequence includes three courses that are taught in the foundation year. In the first course, emphasis is placed on exposing students to theory, and assignments are designed that help students examine developmental and policy issues from a theoretical perspective. Among other authors, students read Cassidy (1999), Saleebey (2006), and Payne (2005) in order to expand fluency with theory and build capacities to interpret client and community material.

A strong theoretical foundation is critical for expanding capacities to interpret cultural material, to evaluate that quality of the attachment to cultural structures, to identify processes associated in negotiating multiple cultures, and to locate culture as one of the core elements that define the human experience.

LESSONS LEARNED: THE SIGNIFICANCE OF CULTURE

Growing up in East Los Angeles with the knowledge that my origins are Mexican and American Indian fostered an early, but undefined and unspoken, awareness of difference. My abilities to make sense of "difference" expanded as my vocabulary and world expanded. I am Chicana, a second generation Mexican American woman, and Oglala. Although the process was/is often painful, I have learned skills that support my abilities to bridge difference and to negotiate social and cultural borders. My work is influenced by my belief that culture is a central and defining element of life. Perhaps, this can be attributed to the fact that my development occurred in a world that was/is saturated with cultural material.

I have been engaged in efforts to understand the influence of cultural material throughout my career. I developed a reference point for discussing evidence that culture endures, that culture is replicated, that culture informs/influences development and identity, and that culture is a resource. I have labeled this reference point: "Lessons from Marrano Beach."

Marrano Beach, also know as El Rancho de Don Daniel, is located in the Los Angeles County region of West San Gabriel Valley, near the intersections of Rosemead and San Gabriel Boulevards. This area is due east of the thriving Los Angeles community that is the historic home of a large Mexican origin population. For years (1930-1970), Marrano Beach was the destination for family outings and social activities for Mexicans/Chicanos living in East Los Angeles and the surrounding communities. It is a touchstone that symbolizes much of the East Los Angeles historical and cultural experience. It has been celebrated in song, in literature, and in the oral histories and folklore of East Los Angeles. Marrano Beach symbolizes the rich cultural inheritance of the Mexican/Latino community and the tenacity and strength of cultural experiences that influence individual and family development.

The title, "Lessons from Marrano Beach" masks emic/insider knowledge. If one knows Marrano Beach, one knows something of the Mexican, Chicano, East Los Angeles experience. Marrano Beach is a shorthand term that alludes to a particular experience for nurturing families/community, for managing racist and discriminatory practices, and for celebrating and practicing values, beliefs, and patterns of behavior. Yet, the lesson from Marrano Beach is universal. We all know and possess "insider" cultural knowledge that comforts, sustains, defines, and challenges. How can social workers access this knowledge, evaluate it and decide whether/how it is integrated in intervention strategies? One lesson from Marrano Beach is the idea that "insider" knowledge is the foundational material from which "culturally appropriate, culturally relevant" interventions are crafted. Another lesson from Marrano Beach indicates that the prevailing paradigms on cultural competency do not adequately explain or examine how/why cultural material resonates across generations. Current conceptualizations on cultural competency can be elaborated by invoking attachment theory in the analysis of individual, family, and community development. Developing knowledge about the bonds that exist between individuals, families, and communities and cultural material can enrich capacities to engage across cultures and to negotiate difference.

Attention to culture and the intersections that link culture, practice, and social justice were relatively limited in the social work curricula of the era when I studied for my MSW degree. Much knowledge about the intersection between culture and social work practice has been gleaned from direct practice with clients, consultation with peers, reflections on process, research, and study. The literature addressing cultural diversity and social work has flourished in the last ten years, and there are some key authors that have influenced my understanding of issues, including Diane de Anda's (1984) work on bicultural socialization, Duran and Duran (1995) on the American Indian postcolonial experience, James Green's (1999) work on ethnographic interviewing, and Renato Rosaldo (1989) and others who work in the area of cultural studies. The literature on the strengths perspective and narrative approaches provided a language for the culturally focused work that was pioneered and has developed since the mid 1970s. I have learned that the examination of culture and analysis of cultural influences on development and behavior must be grounded in theory and the literature. The quality of the knowledge that is required to do culturally focused work requires that social workers engage in constant and rigorous study of issues throughout their professional careers.

Consultation with peers and analysis of practice has played a vital role in advancing understanding of cultural material and context. During my MSW graduate career and since graduation, I engaged with Chicano/a Latino/a and American Indian professionals and other clinicians of color as we struggled to modify what was learned in school in efforts to meet the needs of the clients and communities that we served. We discussed cases, shared resources, collaborated on cases, reflected on practice, experimented with methods and modalities, created organizations, crafted policy recommendations, and designed culturally-based intervention programs. We struggled to figure out how to deliver services in another language, and how to engage families and communities that were not represented in the literature. Consultations always included discussions about the integration of cultural material and historical, political, and social context in the work and about increasing the responsiveness and relevance of service delivery systems. In the early years, we were often the sole Latino/a, American Indian or practitioners of color in the work environment. The intersection of policy, practice, and social justice was always visible in the stories of clients and in the circumstances of their lives. In individual and small group consultations and in organizational meetings, discussions occurred that focused on the need to craft interventions and to transform service delivery systems in order to increase cultural relevance and to address social, health, and educational disparities.

My personal narrative, the narratives of clients, literature reviews, and research findings have affirmed that culture is the focal point of human experience. In this scenario, social workers are always engaging across cultural terrain. Social, political, historical, geographic, sexual, and gendered borders are negotiated and contested as personal and professional life is constructed. From my perspective, the prevailing paradigm on cultural competency can be enriched by examining how/why social workers can cross these borders and this contested psychosocial terrain. Social workers can investigate the strengths and resources as one moves from our world into the world of the "other."

The social work profession articulates a commitment to examine and attend to diversity in standards developed by the National Association of Social Work. The document, Indicators for the Achievement of the NASW Standards for Cultural Competence in Social Work Practice (NASW, 2007), lays out elaborate and eloquent guidelines that provide a roadmap supporting culturally competent practice. The many dimensions of diversity that characterize the U.S., social work ethical principles, clear definitions of terms, and recommendations for engaging in the life long process of developing cultural competency are provided. This author acknowledges the strengths of this document and the commitment of colleagues in the profession who crafted these guidelines for practice. Similar to other discussions on cultural competency, this document tends to be prescriptive. Further, many social workers tend to seek recipes for culturally competent practice. Practitioners can avoid cookie cutter approaches to practice and enhance capacities to engage across cultures by employing a solid theoretical orientation integrated with knowledge of the client's culture and of the social and political context.

In the Los Angeles community, there is a network of social workers who have considered these issues for thirty years. Great strides have been made by way of introducing increasing numbers of Latino/a, African American, Asian and Pacific Islander, and American Indian/Alaska Native students to MSW programs and to the profession. Within the profession and social work education, a more expansive and inclusive analysis of diversity signals that the issue of "difference" is embraced by the profession. However, the numbers of students entering and graduating from doctorate programs in social work do not reflect the demographics of the region. Moreover, the needs of the local community remain relatively unchanged in spite of the increasing number of MSW programs and MSW graduates. Latino/a, African American, Asian and Pacific Islander, and American Indian/Alaska Native populations, continue to experience high rates of poverty, health and educational disparities, community and interpersonal violence and other social problems. (See recent reports by Leory in the Los Angeles Times, Los Angeles County, and United Way Los Angeles). Social policy continues to articulate initiatives that are hostile to poor and vulnerable constituents. The Leave No Child Behind and Temporary Assistance to Needy Families legislation do not appear to have promoted the health and well-being of the community. Immigration reform proposals fall far short of addressing the complexity of this issue in a way that is consistent with the ethics and values of the profession. The question arises: how does the profession examine and meet the needs of culturally diverse populations when social policy and social service delivery systems are hostile and unfavorable to these communities? How is "cultural competence" integrated into social practice under these circumstances? How can one interpret behavior through a cultural lens?

Attachment theory complements and elaborates on prescriptive and prevailing conceptualizations about cultural competency. Practice and research within the American Indian community indicates that individuals, families, and communities "attach" to cultural material in a process that parallels the process that unfolds between infant and caregiver. The outcomes of attachment experiences (to caregiver and/or to culture) are similar and result in feelings of safety, security and trust or insecurity, anxiety or ambivalence. Attachment theory demonstrates utility for examining the quality of the bonds that exist between a people and the complexity and depth of their cultural inheritance. In so doing, the prevailing paradigms on cultural competency are elaborated, because capacities for evaluating the "place/role" of culture in the analysis of issues and the identification of strengths are promoted.

Practice and research provide ample evidence that many American Indians as well as members of other disenfranchised, displaced, and vulnerable poplulations are born into families and communities that are fundamentally shaped by traumatic loss experiences. This population can include survivors of natural disasters, such as Hurricane Katrina, the children and grandchildren of Holocaust survivors and genocides, as well as refugees, immigrants, and families that are marginalized and disenfranchised across generations. Traumatic loss experiences that are unspoken and unexamined may result in a host of negative life circumstances that may or may not be within the control of the individual, family or community. In this circumstance, vulnerabilities for a host of psychosocial and health problems are increased. Historical trauma and the intergenerational transmission of loss can confound grief, mourning, and meaning-making processes. When this occurs, functioning and psychosocial well-being can be affected across generations, resulting in families and communities that are populated by the walking wounded.

Distress is compounded as one negotiates the borders between different cultural worlds. When capacities to negotiate borders are undermined, when abilities to cognitively process the (intergenerational) sources of distress, shame, frustration, rage, and self-doubt can develop.

My research and practice experience indicates that the resources for addressing these issues and for strengthening families and communities are often found within the cultural material of the community. When losses experiences are interpreted, framed, and reorganized, abilities to engage with the world in ways that promote heath and well-being are enhanced. Attachment theory, which offers an explanatory model for interpreting the quality of the bonds that exist between infant and care-giver, can support analysis of the quality of the bonds that exist between cultural structures and individuals, families, and communities, and it can advance understanding of the loss and traumatic experiences that are common to all humanity. My practice and research within the American Indian and Chicano/a Latino/a communities affirm another lesson from Marrano Beach. Cultural material influences the processes of making meaning and integrating the trauma and loss; therefore, a strong theoretical foundation in attachment processes can support the social worker's capacity to understand and interpret behaviors and events from the perspective of the client. Cultural relevance and cross-cultural practice can be promoted by integrating ethnographic and narrative techniques with the theoretical understanding of attachment and loss.

LESSON LEARNED: THE IMPORTANCE OF REFLECTION AND CONSULTATION

I cannot overemphasize the importance of consultation and of self reflection. Social work practice at all levels of practice mixes science with art; practice is an extraordinarily creative, innovative, and flexible process that is supported by a bank of knowledge. I know that I have sometimes felt as if I were "flying by the seat of my pants" or responding instinctually to content/process. However, the capacity to engage at this level is not (nor should it be) an instinctual or free-floating activity. It is predicated on the capacity to "pull up" and integrate knowledge, expertise, and skill in the moment that it is required. This capacity de-velops as one engages in a consistent and rigorous practice of reflecting on the work. This includes examination of personal and professional reactions to the work and participating in an on-going process of cri-tique and evaluation. In practice, it is the "self" that is the medium for the work. Therefore, it is critical to engage in activities that promote the development of the self and promote insight and self-awareness. One must be mindful and aware of the filters that influence the processing of information, the evaluation of information, and the development of interventions.

I recall that early in my career, I was assigned a client who was a monolingual, Spanish-speaking working class man who was referred by the courts for an incident of domestic violence. He reported to the agency with his wife and young child. He proceeded to challenge my credentials, inquiring about my marital status and whether I was married to a Mexican. At the conclusion of the intake, I offered him an appointment (after all, that was a minimum expectation), but I certainly didn't have a favorable impression of him. He irritated me, because he seemed to confirm every negative stereotype of Mexican men. My expectations were low, and much to my surprise, he returned for a second appointment. Eventually, a therapeutic relationship was established, and we actually came to respect one another. What was the barrier to services? I was the barrier. My preconceptions about who he was (entirely false and unfounded), my reactions to his tone and questioning (perfectly within his rights and normal to wonder about the person sitting opposite), and my distaste for his "problem" could have created fundamental obstacles in his ability to meet the mandate of the court. He was ready, I was not. How many clients are "ready" before the social worker? How many times are social workers responsible for a therapeutic failure or the inability of a client to meet mandated expectations? Quite possibly, we are responsible more times than we know for a therapeutic failure. I think that one of the best safeguards to protect against this lies in the ability to consider and reflect upon what we do and to determine why we are doing it. There is a clinical maxim, "Don't ask your client to do something that you are unwilling to do." We cannot ask clients to examine and reflect on their circumstances, if we are unwilling to reflect on ours.

The process of reflecting on practice is closely related to the process of consultation. Often, consultation and supervision are reduced to activities for monitoring paperwork and deadlines. I am referring to the process of examining the work and evaluating interventions, at all levels of practice. This mechanism is critically important in assuring that clients and communities consistently experience a high level of service. Consultation provides the venue for exploring every element of the process, for identifying missteps and successes, for considering why an intervention is appropriate or inappropriate, and for promoting creativity and innovation. Often, the consultative process leads one to identify issues that are broader and of greater magnitude than what was initially apparent. For example, my understanding about the intersection of practice and policy has evolved as a result of work with undocumented clients and the opportunity to "talk" about that work. Certainly, my understanding about the consequences of the Boarding Schools in American Indian/Alaska Native communities and intergenerational loss has expanded as a result of conversations with colleagues, who confronted similar issues. As reported earlier in this essay, my understanding of culture elaborated through consultation. Consultation has provided the opportunity for many "A-ha!" moments, and these moments result in benefits that accrue to clients and constituents. To play on the title of a popular book, "Almost, everything I need to know about social work, I've learned through consultation with colleagues."

A final case example illustrates that theory, culture, reflective practice, and consultation can result in better outcomes for clients and can strengthen the capacities of social workers.

> A Spanish-speaking man from Mexico presented at the agency, requesting information about services for his wife who was "depressed." I provided information about the services available, learned that his wife was willing to come in for an interview and scheduled an intake interview. Both husband and wife came to the appointment, and the wife indicated that she would like her husband to participate in the interview. They were articulate, responsive, and readily engaged with me.
>
> During the course of the intake interview, I learned that they were undocumented, that the journey from their home town to the United States was fraught with danger, that they were living in the area (downtown Los Angeles) without family or a support system for the last several months, and that they were both employed at different factories. They appeared to have a very strong bond, and the wife appeared very sad about their circumstance and unsure that the decision to immigrate was worth the struggle. She did not appear clinically depressed, but she was obviously distressed. The source of her distress was somewhat puzzling; it did not seem that the losses associated with immigration were the sole source of her distress. Although this interview took place about 23 years ago, I still recall the tenderness, concern, and warmth that they exhibited in verbal communication and non-verbal behaviors. We agreed to schedule another meeting in order to explore the losses resulting

from leaving families and their home in Mexico and the challenges associated with building a life in Los Angeles.

The next sessions focused on gathering more history about individual and family development and their life in Mexico, learning about the immigration story, dreams and aspirations, monitoring the wife's mood and functioning, and trying to rule out other conditions. She appeared stable, but there was no dramatic improvement. At the fourth meeting, I learned another reason for the wife's distress. She had been raped by a foreman at the factory shortly after she was hired. She did not initially disclose the rape to her husband. She felt very confused and conflicted, because at one point during the assault, she decided not to resist. She was ashamed and unsure about how her husband would react. She told him about the rape three weeks after it occurred in response to his concerns about why she was "depressed" and "panicky." Her disclosure triggered his request for services, although he did not want to discuss her "condition" until she was ready to introduce the subject.

The clinical work continued for about eleven months after the disclosure. Immediately after the disclosure, two priority issues were addressed: securing a medical evaluation for the wife and finding new employment without jeopardizing the precarious financial realities of their life. The work included individual and conjoint sessions that focused on addressing the trauma, eliciting the immigration story, providing a supportive and collaborative space for them to explore reactions to the immigration journey, reactions to the rape, the meaning of the rape and the degree to which it would influence their relationship, dreams and life, and connecting them with additional resources in the community. The interviews were conducted in Spanish and shared cultural references helped to foster intimacy and served as metaphors in our conversations.

Initially, my clinical supervisor recommended that I refer the wife to the staff psychiatrist for a medication evaluation. Then, when the rape was disclosed, I was encouraged to recommend reporting the rape to law enforcement. My interventions and the couple's behavior raised concerns for my supervisor: why didn't the husband express more rage; why was he intruding on his wife's therapy; was his participation evidence of his need to control and dominate his wife, since he couldn't prevent the rape; was the wife's sad affect evidence of dependent or depressed personality; should they be encouraged to return to Mexico; how could I appropriately respond to two clients with two separate sets of issues; was I idealizing the couple and minimizing their psychological impairments?

I requested permission from my supervisor to consult with colleagues in the community who worked with a similar client population. The questions and directives of my supervisor were within standards of practice. However, the feedback was not always helpful to me as I struggled to remain available and to provide meaningful interventions. Fortunately, my supervisor understood my quandary and approved my request. Consultation with colleagues proved very beneficial in helping me to respond to my supervisor's questions, in clarifying my reactions to my supervisor and the clients, and in developing and evaluating an intervention plan. The consultations with peers provided the opportunity to examine the developmental, cultural, social, political, and legal complexities of the case.

Although the agency would have received a higher reimbursement rate for services if the psychiatrist were involved, the terms of the contract with the Department of Mental Health would have limited treatment options and precluded the husband's involvement. Consultation with peers provided ample opportunities to explore treatment options and the cultural dimensions of client behaviors and client interactions. Some interpretations of behavior could indicate pathology using the prevailing paradigms of the era. However, when viewed through a cultural lens, these same behaviors appeared appropriate and healthy within the context of the clients' experiences. Consultation also provided direction in examining the social and political factors that promoted immigration, as well as the issues that needed to be negotiated in the new community and the losses that are associated with immigration.

Several lessons for practice are embedded in this case. It is critical to disentangle pathology and culture; the responses of both clients made sense when examined through a cultural lens and provided evidence of strength and resilient capacities. The husband's behavior epitomized the Mexican traditional values of stoicism, protection, responsibility, and sacrifice. He *was* angry, guilty, and shamed. However, his overriding concern was to find a way to comfort and protect his wife. His capacity to defer his needs in order to focus on his wife exemplified maturity, integrity, and love.

Responses to trauma are influenced by the pre-existing level of functioning, capacities to make meaning of the traumatic event, and the ability to give voice to the experience. The decision to immigrate to the United States was fueled by a spirit of adventure as well as economic instability in Mexico. The clients had no children; they were young and believed that opportunity awaited them. The clients were relatively well-educated and demonstrated good judgment, insight, and self-awareness. The wife's reactions to the rape were within the range of normal responses. The support that she derived from her spouse and the therapeutic relationship helped her to grieve the experience, consider how the experience affected her current functioning, anticipate future challenges, and reestablish a sense of control and safety.

The legal system may not always be perceived as a resource and protection for clients. The clients were sophisticated enough to understand that the delay in reporting and the wife's return to the factory after the rape undermined any legal protections that might be available. Because of their status as undocumented workers, there were additional concerns that they believed would result in greater vulnerabilities if they spoke with law enforcement.

Clients may experience multiple losses, and losses can accumulate and overwhelm capacities. These clients left families and support systems in Mexico with dreams for a better life and new opportunities as the Mexican economy collapsed. Their dreams quickly developed nightmarish characteristics. They were robbed by the "coyotes" (smugglers) who provided passage across the border. Their standard of living was lower in Los Angeles than in Mexico, and the absence of support systems and friends left them isolated and depleted. They were relatively new to Los Angeles and had not yet established a network to help in negotiating the new environment, and the shame of the rape initially fueled mistrust and apprehension for both. They were compelled to live in fear and on the margins of society as a result of their undocumented status. The aftermath of the rape threatened their very survival. They were on the brink of despair, but strong survival instincts and the quality of their attachment bond promoted capacities to resolve this crisis. They drew upon deeply held cultural values and spiritual beliefs as they struggled to assign meaning to the experience and as they sought to reorganize their life and relationship.

Clients are truly "experts" in their own lives and may possess many strengths and capacities that are not readily apparent. Cultural values, relationship protocols and stories provided support for interventions. Courage and the strength of caring and character provided the impetus for this couple to reach out for assistance. This capacity was humbling and inspirational. At intake, their circumstance was grim and challenging. The process of examining their circumstance was often painful and difficult. At termination, there were indicators that they could successfully negotiate the challenges that still lay before them, and there was a hopeful sense that they could persevere.

CONCLUSION

In this essay, I share some reflections on social work practice and education that are derived from my own practice and scholarship. My own awareness of difference, my experiences negotiating different cultural worlds, and encounters with racism and discrimination influence my efforts to engage in practice that promotes insight, builds capacities, and pursues social justice. The social, historical, and political movements that provided the backdrop for my development have fueled an interest in learning about context. My experience being raised in an environment that was rich with Mexican, Oglala, and East Los Angeles cultural material has stimulated my desire to learn more about the influence of culture and its role in development and on the lived realities of daily life.

I have learned many lessons in over twenty-five years of practice. I have learned of the importance of developing a sound theoretical foundation to support every arena of practice. I know that I need basic understanding of the developmental tasks that are associated with productive functioning in *this* society. I have learned that I need theories that help me investigate and interpret social, historical, and political context and that locate the analysis of culture in a political framework. I have learned about the importance of attachment and that individuals, families, and communities establish bonds and relationships with cultural material that may be as influential as the bonds that infants establish with caregivers and the bonds that unfold across the lifespan. I have learned that reflection and consultation have been invaluable assets supporting my development. I have come to have deep appreciation for strengths and narrative approaches. As I began to read this literature, I found language and structure that explained the work my colleagues and I were engaged in–designing services for populations that are not always visible in the literature. Self-reflection, collaboration and partnerships with colleagues, and consultation have helped me to examine my own experiences, evaluate the circumstances of constituents, and conduct research. I have learned to listen, and I have been informed. These lessons have made me a better parent, spouse, daughter, friend, teacher and social worker. I am grateful to the clients, organizations, mentors, colleagues, and students who have supported my development.

REFERENCES

Cassidy, J., & Shaver, P. R. (1999). *Handbook of attachment: Theory, research and clinical applications*. New York: Guilford Press.

de Anda, D. (1984). Bicultural socialization: Factors affecting the minority experience. *Social Work*, March-April, 101-107.

Duran, B., & Duran, E. (1995). *Native American post-colonial psychology*. New York: State University of New York.

Green, J. W. (1999). *Cultural awareness in human services*. Needham Heights, MA: Allyn & Bacon.

Ledesma, R. (2007). American Indian and Alaska Native Children: A legacy of suffering, survival and strength. In N. Cohen, T. Tran, & S. Rhee (Eds.), *Multicultural approaches in caring for children, youth and their families*, 114-147; Boston: Pearson.

Ledesma, R. (2007). The urban Los Angeles American Indian experience: Notes from the field. *Journal of Ethnic & Cultural Diversity in Social Work*, 16 (1/2), 27-60.

Leovy, J. (2007). Murder Stalks Minorities in The Los Angeles Times, 8-19-2007.

Los Angeles County, Children's Planning Council. (2006). Los Angeles County 2006 Children's ScoreCard.

Neimeyer, R. A. (Ed.) (2002). Meaning Reconstruction and the Experience of Loss, Washington, DC: American Psychological Association.

Payne, M. (2005). *Modern social work theory* (Third Edition). Chicago, Illinois: Lyceum Books.

Rosaldo, R. (1989). *Culture and truth: The remaking of social analysis*. Boston: Beacon Press.

Saleebey, D. (2006). *The strengths perspective in social work practice* (Fourth Edition). Boston: Pearson Education, Inc.

United Way Los Angeles. (2003). A Tale of Two Cities, Bridging the Gap Between Promise and Peril.

United Way Los Angeles and The Urban League. (2005). The State of Black Los Angeles.

Yellow Horse Brave Heart, M., & DeBruyn, L. M. (1998). The American Indian holocaust: Healing historical unresolved grief. *American Indian and Alaska Native Mental Health Research*, 8 (2), 56-78.

Cultural Competence:
An Ethical Requirement

Paula Allen-Meares

INTRODUCTION

Cultural competence is one of the foundations for both social work education and social work practice in the evolving political, social, and economic climates of the day. An increased focus on diversity, an influx of immigrants, and continued political unrest throughout the world are only a few examples of why social workers must be proactive in fulfilling the tenets of the profession that prohibit discrimination and promote the understanding of the differences that make individuals unique.

But how can practitioners fulfill these tenets while simultaneously avoiding the contamination of media, prejudice, and the past? They can do so by understanding history; knowing the guidelines of their professional role; educating themselves about cultures, beliefs, and norms that do not reflect their own; and ultimately examining themselves.

CULTURAL COMPETENCE

In Context

The United States has a rich history of opening its arms to all who wish to call it their home–"Give me your tired, your poor, your huddled masses yearning to breathe free . . ." Due in part to this early open door policy, the country has been metaphorically referred to as a *melting pot*, the underlying concept of which is a sociological model that stresses assimilation. Using a macro focus, the United States declared itself a country where races, cultures, and orientations meet and blend together to form the new identity of *Americans* and adopted the motto *E pluribus unum*, from many we are one.

As we enter the years of the 21st century, the melting pot concept has proven to be an outdated concept in America, reflecting an inaccurate view of our perceptions and attitudes towards race, culture, and personal relationships. Indeed, there has been a shift in focus away from the macro and towards a more micro view, celebrating and upholding those traits, beliefs, and special features that make each of us unique. In this *microcosm* where diversity is prized, we are individuals first and Americans second. The past 30 years have seen diversity celebrated and embraced in the public sentiment, debated and redefined in political circles, and argued in the highest courts.

Increasingly, social conditions, political climates, economic situations, and religious beliefs have placed the *microcosm* under the powerful lens of public opinion and scrutiny. As a country, we have decided that those traits, practices, or beliefs that make each individual unique amongst a sea of fellow countrypersons not only makes each special, but also highlights that we are often very different from one another. As a result, this country has seen feats of amazing strength and healing in commonalities, as well as shocking instances of intolerance and violence in misunderstanding and suspicion.

This is the conflicted context in which social workers practice and the environment that contributes to one of the paradoxes of the profession. As practitioners, social workers must take special care to reject stereotypical socialization, both explicit and implicit, and the negative effects of social conditions (racism, homophobia, sexism, etc.) on their professional behavior and judgment. Simultaneously, social workers must provide professional services to individuals or groups who have been negatively affected by those same social conditions. As difficult as it is to work within this context, social workers must take great care not to place restrictions or assumptions on those who are depicted in negative terms or devalued because of their unique characteristics, but to give precedence to professional responsibility rather than personal beliefs or society's efforts to contaminate perception. In fact, to be truly effective, social workers must become sensitized to the role culture plays in our lives, and practice the skills necessary to address issues that may arise in a cultural context.

In our 1992 article "Is Social Work Racist?" (McMahon & Allen-Meares, 1992), my co-author and I agreed with Gallegos' (1984) statement that "social work practitioners who lack the skill, attitudes, and knowledge to work effectively in cross-cultural settings are incompetent" (p. 1), a sentiment with which I still agree. Given the objectives of the profession, knowledge and skills in cultural competence are imperative. The idea of combining the macro-level unity of the melting pot with the appreciation of the microcosm of celebrated diversity may be a superficial goal for others, but for social workers it is a sincere objective, and cultural competence is an important benchmark in achieving that goal.

The Council for Social Work Education (CSWE), the standard bearer for schools of social work accreditation, indicates that one of social work education's purposes includes "preparing social workers to practice without discrimination, with respect, and with knowledge and skills related to clients' age, class, color, culture, disability, ethnicity, family structure, gender, marital status, national origin, race, religion, sex, and sexual orientation," and charges that graduates must demonstrate ability to practice in such a manner, as it is one of the specific purposes of the social work profession (Council for Social Work Education, 2001, p. 5). Under the heading of *Values and Ethics*, CSWE also includes educating students in diversity issues, stressing that such content "emphasizes the interlocking and complex nature of culture and personal identity" (Council for Social Work Education, 2001, p. 9).

The National Association of Social Workers (NASW), the regulating body for social work standards and ethics, takes this concept a step further. The *Code of Ethics* (NASW, 1999) states that one clear goal for the practitioner is to be sensitive to cultural and ethnic diversity through experience and study. The *Code* calls for competence in recognizing the strengths within cultures and the differences that make races and cultures unique. With this as a professional directive, it logically follows that not only is the lack of cultural competence and sensitivity contrary to the principles of social work, it is, in fact, unethical.

Discrimination vs. Racial and Cultural Sensitivity

It should be self-evident that discrimination in social work is not only contrary to the very tenets of the profession (i.e., service, social justice, compassion, assistance, human interaction and relationships, and positive change), but discrimination is also patently unethical according to the *Code of Ethics*. Standard 4.02 states, "Social workers should not practice, condone, facilitate, or collaborate with any form of discrimination on the basis of race, ethnicity, national origin, color, sex, sexual orientation, age, marital status, political belief, religion, or mental or physical disability" (1999).

With a specific and established prohibition against most forms of discrimination (gender discrimination being noticeably absent), it follows that one way to combat discrimination in social work practice, as well as in the larger society, is by becoming culturally and racially competent. Standard 1.05 states

(a) Social workers should understand culture and its function in human behavior and society, recognizing the strengths that exist in all cultures.

(b) Social workers should have a knowledge base of their clients' cultures and be able to demonstrate competence in the provision of services that are sensitive to clients' cultures and to differences among people and cultural groups.

(c) Social workers should obtain education about and seek to understand the nature of social diversity and oppression with respect to race, ethnicity, national origin, color, sex, sexual orientation, age, marital status, political belief, religion, and mental or physical disability.

Culture: Why Is It Important?

Culture is often explained utilizing a group of related concepts. Merriam-Webster (n.d.) holds that culture may be defined as "the customary beliefs, social forms, and material traits of a racial, religious, or social group; *also*: the characteristic features of everyday existence . . . shared by people in a place or time" (n.p.). Note that culture embraces the notions of race, national origin, ethnicity, and religious practice.

So why, beyond common respect for the individual, should practitioners sensitize themselves to the differences that people bring with them? First, norms, beliefs, and acceptable behaviors can differ amongst cultures. Some, for example, may find women in the workforce perfectly acceptable, while other cultures could not conceive of a role for women outside of motherhood. This viewpoint is perfectly acceptable but may cause conflict in individuals or between groups.

Additionally, culture is rarely a merely passive part of an individual's life. Culture is an integral part of a person's understanding of self, and any injury or insult to this understanding, even unintentionally, has the potential for harm. Therefore, it is in the best interest of the practitioner to develop an understanding and an appreciation for different cultures that he or she may work with in order to better understand the people themselves.

Reamer (1998) points out that culture often dictates how people react to situations or one another, cope with mental illness, consider the use of drugs, and deal with death. Reamer continues, highlighting that those cultural factors may influence the way social services are provided to community members, or may even influence whether members of certain cultural groups seek services to start with. Reactions or overreactions may be explained by a cultural history, previous experiences, or cultural nuances.

Professional Competence

NASW defines cultural competence as:

> the process by which individuals and systems respond respectfully and effectively to people of all cultures, languages, classes, races, ethnic backgrounds, religions, and other diversity factors in a manner that recognizes, affirms, and values the worth of individuals, families, and communities and protects and preserves the dignity of

each . . . [and a] set of congruent behaviors, attitudes, and policies that come together in a system or agency or among professionals and enable the system, agency, or professionals to work effectively in cross-cultural situations. (NASW, 2001)

The encompassing concept of cultural competence has taken on increased importance within the profession as the understanding of diversity issues and cultural norms within social work has evolved. The 1996 version of the NASW *Code of Ethics* was the first to include the standard for competence in this area, while the NASW board adopted specific standards for cultural competence in 2001. With the rise in immigration and religious and racial-based discrimination, as well as the legalization or illegalization of diversity at both the state and federal levels, it will continue to be a growing factor as social workers assist with immigration, acculturation (a blending of cultures), assimilation (the gradual loss of one culture in favor of another), and cultural understanding and acceptance.

At its core, the call for cultural competence and sensitivity to diversity is another way to emphasize that social workers should focus their attention on those with whom they interact, leaving their own prejudices at the door and respecting differences. But more than this sensitivity to culture is an opportunity to learn about the community in which one works–including not only the people, but also the political, religious, and social nuances that grow from or in response to different cultural influences.

By increasing their sensitivity and awareness, social workers can be in the position to provide people with the services they need or to educate others about people within the culture. For example, if Jorge, an American from a Latino background, and Sami, an American born to Pakastani parents, are in a schoolyard fight, the school social worker may sit down with their parents, explaining to Jorge's parents that while Sami did indeed throw the first jab, it was because Jorge had unknowingly said something offensive–that Sami was a member of one culture when he was in reality a member of another. The two cultures had a shared history of war and oppression, and Sami felt the need to defend his own community. Similarly, if Joanne comes into a social work therapist's office and has an issue with her boss–who continually makes comments about why Joanne, who adheres to a specific religion that considers Monday sacred, cannot work on Mondays–it important for the social worker to understand the context in which the comments are being made.

A Strengths Perspective

Much of the literature discussing cultural competence highlights that a practitioner should consider the very strengths of a culture, especially since those elements that differ from the norm or from those of the majority are often considered bad or wrong. Cultural strengths may come in the form of positive protective skills (Bowman, 2006), the focus on the family, or the belief in higher education and achievement. In effect, clinicians empower their clients through their own beliefs, skills, and relationships (Lee, 2003).

Cultural strengths may also come into play when interacting with someone who is from a minority culture or who is multi-cultural. McAdoo (1993) points out that some may have "cultural myopia" (p. 5), a lack of awareness of their own culture or cultural strengths. This may affect individuals when they do not recognize that there are differences between their personal culture and the culture of others, or when a deeper understanding of their personal cultural influences could serve as a positive influence in their life. Culture may play a large role in self-awareness and self-determination, and the social worker should examine whether this might assist with improving the person's situation.

Cultural Competence and Emerging Social Issues

The influx of new immigrants to the United States presents social workers with both unique opportunities and challenges. According to the Department of Homeland Security (2005), 1,112,373 people from other countries were granted legal resident status. Additionally, 53,813 refugees were documented and 25,257 applications for asylum were received by the federal government. All bring with them their own experiences, beliefs, cultural traits, habits, rituals, and even dress. They carry the opportunity to contribute their perspective to the enrichment of the larger American culture. They also carry their own burdens and sometimes the physical scars of war, disease, or oppression. Social workers have the opportunity to provide direct assistance and services to the immigrant population itself, as well as to those who have spent time in the States–whether born or bred–by way of education and understanding about those who are considered different from their own cultural norms.

In addition, America is also currently dealing with two very pressing and urgent matters that affect all Americans regardless of skin color, gender, or national origin: health care and aging. As the needs of our rapidly aging society increase, and as health care continues to be plagued with ethical debates and costs that put it out of reach for many, cultural factors may come into play on a much larger scale.

At a basic level, it is important for social workers in the geriatric field to understand the cultural norms communities may hold regarding the aging process, caregiving, and the process of death and mourning. It will also become vital for healthcare workers to educate themselves on those topics and others, including beliefs about organ transplant, termination of pregnancy, blood transfusions, and other often pressing and delicate matters. It is also quite crucial that social workers have enough of a knowledge base that they do not associate one set of beliefs with the wrong cultural group–for instance, mistaking one religious group's belief not to seek medical treatment at all (instead relying on prayer) for another religious group's belief that forbids blood transfusions. Not only are the results potentially insulting, they may have dire consequences in healthcare situations.

Nuance may also play a role in social work's response to the social violence that has plagued the United States since the 9/11 terrorist attacks. Based solely on the race, ethnicity, and religion of some of those involved, Americans and American immigrants who merely hold some of the same physical traits, clothing styles, or religious beliefs have found themselves targets of misplaced anger, resentment, and discrimination. Understanding the differences (in addition to the obvious one that all people of a certain race, etc., do not speak or act for all others) between cultures, beliefs, dress, and practices may assist social workers in helping the individual work through his or her own issues, educate and inform others, or contribute to the larger social dialogue regarding these issues.

How Can We Fulfill the Mandate?

With the professional imperative to interact with all people as individuals rather than the sum of their traits or beliefs, how can social workers realistically avoid bringing their own past experiences, their own perceptions, and even their own misinformation with them into a professional situation? Have the governing bodies created a standard that is ultimately unachievable?

March (2004) states that we, as social workers, know that "at its core, culturally competent practice goes far beyond the recognition that we work with colleagues and clients whose backgrounds and experiences may be different from our own" (p. 5). She states that cultural competence includes three elements: self-assessment, lifelong cultural education, and, in turn, cultural advocacy. So when and where do we begin incorporating these three elements into our professional lives?

The institutionalization of the call for cultural competence within social work education is a place for us to start. Here, educators can provide some groundwork for students on theories, issues, and emerging research on diversity, rising social issues, and cultural competence. The University of Michigan School of Social Work, for example, has implemented programming informally titled "PODS," which stands for Privilege, Oppression, Diversity, and Social Justice. The school has incorporated elements of PODS into practice area concentration courses and field practica, and considers PODS "a lens through which the course topics are viewed and critiqued" (University of Michigan School of Social Work, 2005, n.p.). The decision to infuse PODS throughout the curriculum was based on both the mission of the school and the underlying values and objectives of social work; PODS is used as a vehicle to highlight the end goal of social justice for all populations social workers serve.

Reamer (1998) suggests that practitioners can get involved in many events and organizations that will assist them in educating and sensitizing themselves to cultural strengths and issues–for example, keeping up-to-date with the professional literature and continuing education opportunities, as well as getting involved in professional, community, or international groups that organize and sponsor events promoting culture, diversity, and understanding (e.g., NAACP, Oxfam, National Council of LaRaza, ACLU, the National Congress of American Indians).

It is also important for individuals to look within themselves, examining their own concepts of privilege, experiences with racism, and underlying perceptions of themselves and others that they have gathered over time. The process of self-awareness, as an individual and as a practitioner, will evolve with reflection, experience, and continued education. It is here that the answer to the question "How can we fulfill this mandate?" may ultimately rest–we fulfill it in the conscious decisions and self-discovery we make on a regular basis.

REFERENCES

Bowman, P. J. (2006). Considerations role strain and adaptation issues in the strength-based model: Diversity, multilevel, and life-span. *The Counseling Psychologist, 34,* 118.

Council for Social Work Education. (2001). *Educational policy and accreditation standards.* Alexandria, VA: Author.

Department of Homeland Security. (2005). *Yearbook of immigration statistics*. Retrieved March 16, 2007, from http://www.dhs.gov/ximgtn/statistics/publications/yearbook.shtm

Gallegos, J. S. (1984). The ethnic competence model for social work education. In B. W. White (Ed.), *Color in a white society* (pp. 1-9). Silver Spring, MD: National Association of Social Workers.

Lee, M. Y. (2003). A solution-focused approach to cross-cultural clinical social work practice: Utilizing cultural strengths. *Families in Society, 84*(3), 385.

March, J. C. (2004). Social work in a multicultural society. *Social Work, 49*(1), 5.

McAdoo, H. P. (1993). *Family ethnicity: Strength in diversity*. Newbury Park, CA: Sage.

McMahon, A., & Allen-Meares, P. (1992). Is social work racist? A content analysis of recent literature. *Social Work, 37*(6), 533.

Merriam-Webster Online Dictionary. (n.d.). Retrieved March 6, 2007, from http://209.161.33.50/dictionary/culture

National Association of Social Workers. (1999). *NASW code of ethics*. Washington, DC: Author. Retrieved March 5, 2007, from http://www.socialworkers.org/pubs/code/code.asp

National Association of Social Workers. (2001). *NASW standards for cultural competence in social work practice*. Retrieved March 20, 2007, from http://www.socialworkers.org/sections/credentials/cultural_comp.asp.

Reamer, F. G. (1998). In H. P. McAdoo (Ed.), *Ethical standards in social work: A critical review of the NASW Code of Ethics* (pp. 3-14). Newbury Park: Sage.

University of Michigan School of Social Work. (2005). PODS questions and answers: Definitions, history, and scope of PODS. Retrieved March 19, 2007, from http://ssw.umich.edu/orientation/readings/PODSqA.pdf

REFLECTIONS ON THE CHANGING DEMOGRAPHICS AND DIVERSITY "WITHIN"

Latino Population Growth, Characteristics and Language Capacities: Implications for Society, Services and Social Justice

Ramon M. Salcido

INTRODUCTION

At an October 2006 presentation at the Laval University School of Social Service in Quebec, I presented the latest Census information regarding the growth of the Latino/a population in the United States. Quebec is a French-speaking province in Canada with a political concern with French language rights (Kertzer & Arel, 2002). The Quebecois faculty asked for general information about Latino/as with an emphasis on language use, population growth, and the impact on social work education.

Canadian statistics show Canadian Latinos to be about 216,975 (5.5%) and concentrated in the provinces of Ontario and Quebec (Salcido & Ornelas, 2005). Some of the issues presented at this School will be used as topics for stimulating discussion and critical thinking concerning Latinos/as.

The purpose of this paper is to identify social demographic issues about Latinos, using the findings of the available bicentennial Census reports, the 2005 American Community Survey, and the Pew Hispanic Center census tallies. Even though the mid decade 2005 American Community Survey differs from the bicentennial Census in method and population sample, most of the questions are similar to the bicentennial. The combined reports are used to provide insights and speculative trends for stimulating discussion about Latinos. The term Latino in this paper is used to describe anyone from a Hispanic heritage and used here to signify both genders, Latinas (females) and Latinos (males). The designation Hispanic/Latino was created by the federal government in the late 1970s as a category to specify a separate ethnic group. On the other hand, the term Hispanic also has colonial implications because of its derivation from the word Spain (Salcido & Maldonado, 2005). Interestingly, many Latinos also prefer to call themselves by other terms that indicate national origins.

LATINO POPULATION

One in every seven Americans is Latino, according to the data released by the United States Census Bureau (2005). Latinos continue to be the fastest-growing ethnic group in America and account for more than 41.8 million of the 288.3 million people living in the United States.

The U.S. Latino population grew between 1990 and 2000 climbing from 22.4 million in 1990 to 35.3 million in 2000. Furthermore, the population grew again from 35.3 million in 2000 to 41.8 million in 2005, suggesting a fifteen year growth trend. The growth trend is important as it affects most of the regions of America. The population estimates now indicate the Latino population group is now the largest minority ethnic group in the United States. In addition to the growth trend, the social demographics characteristics of this ethnic group merit attention.

What Are the Characteristics of Latinos?

Latinos reflect a variety of national backgrounds and heritage. In relation to heritage, about (58.5%) indicate Mexican background, followed by Puerto Rican (9.6%), Central American (4.8%); Cuban (4.8%) and (2.2%) South American (Guzman, 2001). In addition, many Latinos are foreign born with over 40 percent having nativity outside the United States. Specifically, of the 41.9 million Latinos, about 16.7 million (40%) are foreign born and 25.1 million (60%) native born, suggesting a more than half native born ethnic group (http://www.census.gov).

The U.S. Census Bureau News release reports that the median age of the Latino population to be 27.2 years as compared to 40.4 years for non-Hispanic White population. Of Latino households, 49% are married couples, 19% maintained by a woman with no husband, and about 16% live alone. The release also reports that 60% of Latinos age 25 and over were at least high school graduates, and about 12% had a bachelor's degree or higher. In addition, about 78% of the Latino household population five years and over speak a language other than English at home (http://www.census.gov). The poverty rate for Latinos was about 22.4% compared to 13.3% for the general population, suggesting higher poverty rates (http://www.census.gov).

What About Regional Growth and Residence?

Table 1 demonstrates that since 1990, the four regions have experienced a fifteen year Latino population growth. The combined bicentennial Census estimates and American Community Survey findings suggest there were changes in the Latino population from 1990 to 2000 and 2000 to 2005. Every region experienced population growth, some more than others, over the decade and the fifteen year time period, suggesting a continuous growth pattern. In addition, Latinos appear to be more diffused in

TABLE 1. Regional Distribution & Change of Latino Population,
1990, 2000, & 2005

Region	1990 Distribution #	2000 Distribution #	2005 Distribution #	1990-2000 Change #	2000-2005 Change #
Northeast	3,754,389	5,524,087	5,840,941	1,398,023	316,261
Midwest	1,726,509	3,124,532	3,756,348	1,499,698	631,816
South	6,767,021	11,586,696	14,334,439	4,819,675	2,747,743
West	10,106,140	15,340,503	17,938,975	5,234,363	2,598,472

Region	1990 Distribution %	2000 Distribution %	2005 Distribution %	1990-2000 Change %	2000-2005 Change %
Northeast	7.7%	8.9%	13.9%	8.1%	5.7%
Midwest	16.8%	14.9%	9.0%	39.9%	20.2%
South	30.3%	32.8%	34.2%	71.2%	23.7%
West	45.2%	43.5%	42.8%	51.8%	16.9%

Source: U.S. Census Bureau, 1990 Summary and 2000 Summary, Guzman (2001).
    U.S. Census Bureau, 2005 American Community Survey, General Demographic
    Characteristics: 2005.

their geographic distribution, as some have moved from the traditional Southwestern region to other regions of the country, suggesting population shifts (Guzman & McConnell, 2002; Passel & Zimmerman, 2000).

The 1990 and 2000 Census data, as well as the 2005 American Community Survey show that the West (42.8%) and South regions (34.2%) combined (78%) have the largest proportion of Latinos residing in the United States. The proportion of Latinos living in the Midwest and West decreased continuously between 2000 and 2005, but the percentage of Latinos living in the South and Northeast increased during the same time period, suggesting greater population shifts in these two regions. The analysis supports the argument that Latinos are moving in large numbers into the South and other parts of the country (Therrien & Ramirez, 2002).

The traditional regional areas of settlement have been in the states of the Southwest (see Table 1). The Census data suggest that over the past 15 years, Latinos continue to settle in new regions of the country. Latino immigrants have been attracted to new areas of the country and to mid-sized cities and small towns (Vidal de Haymes & Kilty, 2007). A recent study by the League of United Latin American Citizens indicates that 42% of Latinos reside in suburban areas and small towns not accustomed to large Latino immigrant settlement influxes (League of United American Citizens [LULAC], 2003; Vidall de Haymes & Kilty, 2007).

What About State Population Distribution and Growth?

As noted in Table 1, Latinos are mostly concentrated in the South and West regions of the United States. In 2005, more than half of the country's Latinos resided in the states of California (12.5 million), Texas (7.8 million), and Florida (3.4 million). Using the Latino population counts tabulated for each state by the Pew Hispanic Center tabulations, the top ten states showing high population growth changes from 2000 to 2005 were identified (http://pewhispanic.org). States having over 50 percent growth were: North Dakota (62.1%), Arkansas (58.6%), South Carolina (51.4%), and Tennessee (51.3%). Furthermore, states with a 40 percent change range were: Nevada (43.%), North Carolina (48.2%), Georgia (47%); Alabama (40.3%) and Mississippi (41.3%). The tabulations show that more states in the Southern region experienced higher Latino population increases when compared to any of the other states. One explanation for the recent Latino migration to these states is that these states have tight labor markets and a new service economy in the Sun Belt (Vidal de Haymes & Kitty, 2007).

What About Language Capacity and Bilingualism?

The 2005 American Community Surveys, as in the 1990 and 2000 Censuses, asked persons aged 5 and over if they spoke a language other than English at home. The persons who answered "yes" were also asked to indicate how well they spoke English. Persons who spoke English "very well" were considered to have no difficulty with English. However, those who indicated they spoke English "well," "not well," or "not at all," were considered to have difficulty with English (Census, 2005; Shin & Bruno, 2003).

The 2005 American Community Survey findings report that of the over 37 million of the U.S. Latino residents five years of age or older, 29 million (78%) spoke Spanish at home. Specifically, of the 20.7 million native born Latinos, about 13.1 million (64%) spoke Spanish. On the other hand, of the 16.6 million foreign born Latinos, 15.8 (96%) speak Spanish at home, indicating higher use of Spanish by immigrants than native born Latinos.

A Census indicator of bilingualism is the proportion of persons from the Census data who respond that they speak their ethnic language at home while also reporting that they speak English very well (see Table 2). The 2005 Survey showed that of the Latino population over five, 8.1 million (21.7%) speak only English and that 29 million

TABLE 2. Latino Language Capacities Age 5 and Over

	Population	Subgroup %	Subgroup %
All U.S. Latinos	37,346,131	100.0	
Speak only English	8,131,764	21.7	
Speak Spanish	29,073,428	77.8	100.0
English very well	14,417,684		9.5
English well	5,559,872		19.10
English not well	5,616,346		19.30
English not at all	3,479,526		11.96
Speak other language	140,939		0.04

Sources: U.S. Census Bureau, 2005 American Community Survey.
NOTE: B16006. Language Spoken at home by ability to speak English for the population 5 years and over (Hispanic or Latino) (http://www.census.gov).

(78%) speak Spanish, suggesting more Latinos to be Spanish speakers than English speakers. However, of the subgroup that is Spanish speaking, 14. 4 million (49.6%) speak "English very well," suggesting close to half of the Spanish speaking subgroup are bi-lingual. On the other hand, if one adds those who spoke "English well," 5.5 million (19.3%), with those who spoke "English very well" (19.2%), the combined figure becomes about 68%, suggesting a high percentage are bilingual and acculturating, not assimilating, into U.S. society.

IMPLICATIONS

In conclusion, in this essay, a number of demographic trends in the Latino population have been described on both national and regional levels. These social demographics merit attention as these trends have ramifications for social work and social work educators.

Societal Level

The Latino population is young with a large family size and has poverty rates higher than the rest of the population. Many Latinos are foreign-born and Spanish-speaking. Among the most salient issues is the ethnic population growth in the regions and country, the large numbers of Latinos who speak Spanish, and the high percentage who are bilingual. One explanation for this growth has been high levels of migration by immigrant Latinos from Mexico, Central and South America. The increase has become a catalyst for anti-immigrant racist attitudes toward both foreign born immigrants and native born Latinos. The most observable reaction has been the dramatic increase in public opposition to undocumented persons immigrating to the United States and speaking in Spanish, resulting in an English-only movement. Another is blaming the immigrants for contributing to neighborhood decay, poverty, and the draining of social services.

Another manifestation of this perspective is the demand that Latinos assimilate, like the rest of the other ethnic immigrant groups in the U.S., and speak English. However, Crawford (1992) claims that linguistic assimilation to English is faster than before, with the exception of communities that were incorporated by the U.S., such as Puerto Rico and communities in the Southwest. Our analysis shows that Latinos are moving toward bilingualism not Spanish only. According to our analysis, 72% of Latinos are Spanish-speaking, and of this language group, over 60% speak English "very well" and "well" suggesting a high percentage of bilinguals. These observational trends promise to be more pronounced in many areas of the countries. More studies are needed on language shifts and maintenance.

Service Level

Social workers and their service organizations face a number of challenges in dealing with Latino demographic growth and language issues. On a service level, demographic issues require that social workers strive to develop culturally competent services for Latinos, both native and immigrant. The existence of culturally and linguistically sensitive programs is important in servicing the needs of Latinos. One major strategy social service agencies can pursue is to hire bilingual social workers who have professional experience in working with Latinos. Another strategy is to offer training to aid their staff in developing cross-cultural skills. Finally, social service agencies can initiate efforts to subsidize Spanish language acquisition for social workers who are seeking to become bilingual and gain professional experience in working with immigrant and native Latinos.

Social Justice Level

As Latinos follow economic opportunities to traditional and new areas of the country, they may encounter anti-immigrant attitudes and racist practices including institutional racism (Martinez-Brawly & Paz Martinez-Brawly, 2001.) The anti-immigrant sentiment calls for an active response on the part of social workers and social work academic programs. Social work practitioners and educators can join with immigrant rights organizations to promote national policies that move toward the achievement of social justice, including culturally competent social work practice. The existence of social justice actions is contingent upon the knowledge and skills of social workers. Therefore, social work education programs will need to respond to these demographic issues and develop teaching strategies for implementing a multicultural curriculum that incorporates Latino content and social activism.

In my opinion, social work educators are becoming more concerned with research funding and teaching students how to change the client, than in social justice and actions for the rights of Latino immigrants and the poor. Unfortunately, we risk teaching our students to become like elites, only concerned with their own class interests and being social control agents, but not learning how to advocate for the under classes such as the immigrant poor.

REFERENCES

Crawford, J. (1992). Hold your tongue: Bilingualism and the politics of English only. Reading, Mass: Addison-Wesley.

Guzman, B., & McConnell, E. D. (2002). The Hispanic population: 1990-2000 growth and change. *Population Research and Policy Review*, Vol. 21: 109-128.

Ketzer, D. I., & Arel, D. (2002). Census and identity: The politics of race, ethnicity, and language in national censuses. Cambridge University Press: London.

League of United Latin American Citizens. (2003). LULAC outlines a vision of America as Hispanic population grows. Retrieved March 3, 2007from website: http:www. LULAC.org.

Martinez-Brawley, E. E. & Paz Martinez-Brawley, Z. (2002). Immigrants, refugees and asylum seekers: The challenge of services in the Southwest. *Journal of Ethnic & Cultural Diversity in Social Work*, 10 (3), 49-67.

Passel, J. S., & Zimmerman, W. (2000). Are immigrants leaving California? Paper presented at the Annual Meetings of the Population Association of America. Los Angeles, CA.

Pew Hispanic Center. (2006 September). A statistical portrait of Hispanics mid-decade. Table 10. Hispanic Population by State: 2000 and 2005. Retrieved from March 3, 2007 from website: www.pewhispanic.org/reports/middledecade.

Salcido, R. M., & Maldonado, C. (2005). Cross-Cultural practice with Latino clients. Private Practice Section Connection. *NASW*: Washington, DC. Summer.

Salcido, R. M., & Ornelas, V. (2005). Poverty & social justice section connection. *NASW*: Washington, DC. Summer.

Shin, H. B., & Bruno, R. (2003). Language use and English-speaking ability: 2000. *U.S. Department of Commerce Economics and Statistics Administration.* Washington, DC: U.S. Government Printing Office.

Therrien, M., & Ramirez, R. R. (2002). The Hispanic population in the United States. (Current Population Report No. P200535). Washington, DC: U.S. Government Printing Office.

U.S. Census Bureau. Hispanic population passes 40 million. Retrieved June 9, 2005 from website:http://www.census.gov/PressRelease/www/reseases/archives/population/005164html.

U.S. Census Bureau. New population profiles released by Census Bureau American Community Survey Data Iterated by Race. Retrieved March 04, 2007 from website: http://www.census.gov/Press-Release/www/releases/archives/American community survey.

U.S. Census Bureau. American fact finder [AFF] survey: 2005 American Community Survey. S0201. Selected Population Profile in the United States. Hispanic or Latino (of any race). Retrieved March 3, 2007 from website: http//factfinder.census.gov.

U.S. Census Bureau. American fact finder [AFF], survey: 2005 American Community Survey. B160051. Nativity by Language Spoken at Home by Ability to Speak English for the Population 5 Years and over (Hispanic or Latino) Retrieved March 3, 2007 from website: http//factfinder.census.gov.

Vidal de Haymes., & Kilty, K. M. (2007). Latino population growth, characteristics and settlement trends. *Journal of Social Work Education.* 43. No. 1. Winter, 101-116.

A Nation of Immigrants:
A Call for a Specialization
in Immigrant Well-Being

David W. Engstrom
Amy Okamura

INTRODUCTION

At the turn of the 21st century, social workers increasingly find themselves working with immigrant and refugee clients. Because of historical circumstances, social work developed and solidified its models of
practice and fields of specialization without much regard to the challenges that immigrants face in a new country. This essay contends that
the scope and volume of contemporary immigration require a reexami-
nation of how the profession serves immigrants, including their families
and communities. We argue that social work must develop a new field
of specialization that focuses on and addresses the unique features of the
immigrant experience.

Social work largely came of age in a period of remarkably low immigration to the United States (1920s to the 1960s). As social work began to professionalize in the 1920s, its Progressive-Era concern over immigrant welfare receded. Instead, it operated in a political and social climate that emphasized "Americanization" and total assimilation as the ideal. By the late 1940s and early 1950s, social workers interacted less with first-generation immigrants and more with their children and grandchildren. Indeed, these later generations, comprised largely of European stock, informed much of our initial conceptualization of the processes of assimilation and acculturation. By the late 1960s, less than 5 percent of the country's population was foreign born, the lowest percentage in 120 years. It is not surprising, then, that by the 1960s the need to understand and address the immigrant experience had been pushed to the margins of social work education and practice.

Much has changed over the past 40 years to make immigrants once again central to social work. Starting with large-scale refugee flows in the 1960s and 1970s and immigration fostered by the 1965 Immigration Act (and its subsequent reform), tens of millions of people have come to the United States. These newcomers appear significantly different from their European-born immigrant predecessors in race, skin color, culture, language, and religion. Moreover, immigrants are dispersing into states and communities with little historic experience in receiving newcomers: The states with the fastest growing immigrant populations are mostly in the South. Individuals and families emigrating from Mexico, the Philippines, China, Somalia, and Iraq, to name a few, have not only diversified our society, but also challenged our social services and social work practice.

SOCIAL WORK WITH IMMIGRANTS: RECONSIDERATIONS

The discussion of immigrants and social work requires serious reconsideration. Contemporary social work is organized around fields of specialization such as child welfare, aging, and mental health, which were developed and solidified in an era of little immigration. Although current specializations have much merit for mainstream populations and problems, they nevertheless have limited utility for informing practice with immigrants and refugees, who often require a more holistic and comprehensive approach. Immigrants and refugees have needs that exceed the confines and treatment philosophies of social work and the institutions (such as social services, health care, and education) in which it is practiced.

Most social welfare institutions operate around a set of *sub rosa* mainstream assumptions. To begin with, institutions assume that clients have a general capacity to communicate in English. Institutions assume that clients understand the purpose of programs and services and the laws and regulations that govern their operation. Institutions assume that clients will know how to access information about services, including being able to negotiate the ubiquitous technological innovations such as automated telephone directories and Web-based information. Moreover, institutions assume that clients understand and share basic assumptions about service delivery, such as appointments, referrals, and waiting lists. Institutions assume that clients have already been socialized into knowing their roles and the roles and boundaries of service providers. Finally, institutions assume that clients know their rights and have the capacity to protect their interests by using appeal processes and other due-process procedures.

Immigrants and refugees often find that their interactions with modern and bureaucratic social institutions take the form of cultural collisions (Fadiman, 1998). This is largely because social institutions operate under a different worldview than that to which many immigrants and refugees are accustomed. Moreover, it is assumed that newcomers must accommodate the institutional norms, rather than vice versa. To make these interactions even more problematic, all immigrants and refugees deal with culture shock, acculturation stress, and the difficulty of surviving in a foreign land with little public support. Some newcomers (mostly, but not exclusively refugees) must also deal with experiences of persecution, oppression, and trauma accrued in their country of origin and during migration.

Social workers are theoretically in an ideal position to ease the transition of immigrants to their new land. Few other professions have as a core element one so ideally suited to assist immigrants as the concept of person-in-the-environment, which can easily be extended to include family. Few other professions tightly embrace empowerment and self-determination as guiding principles. Few other professions feature the micro-to-macro range of practice that is tailor-made to address the multiple needs of immigrants. Certainly, few other professions place as much emphasis on cultural competency. In and of themselves, however, these principles are necessary, but not sufficient, for effective work with immigrants and refugees.

Social workers must have a firm grasp of assimilation and acculturation theories to ground their work with immigrants and immigrant families. These theories highlight intergenerational issues experienced by immigrants and zero in on such phenomena as role reversals and conflicts related to their experience of displacement/change. The straight-line assimilation theory used to explain the incorporation of European immigrants has largely been replaced by theories that emphasize the heterogeneity of the assimilation experience and disparate outcomes based on human and social capital. Equally important, contemporary theory does not assume as fact or as a goal that immigrants must shed their culture to live and succeed in the United States. As Andrew Greeley (2006, p. 8) has stated, "They don't have to be like us. They are entitled to be 'strange.' Just as the rest of us are."

In working with immigrants, social workers need to be aware that many immigrant families are composed of members with different immigration statuses (e.g., citizen, legal immigrant, undocumented). Fix and Zimmerman classify these as mixed-status families and estimate that they make up 9 percent of U.S. families (2001). The typical mixed-status family is composed of U.S.-born children with at least one immigrant parent, who may or may not have legal immigration status. These different statuses bring with them varying rights and privileges, among the most important of which are eligibility for government benefits and ability to sponsor family members to immigrate to the United States.

There is another central issue that social workers must be acutely aware of in working with immigrant families. The act of emigration often means that only some family members make the journey to the

United States, leaving others behind to emigrate later. The consequence of this is that many immigrant families are not wholly constituted (and this is true for both legal and unauthorized immigrants). Legal immigration frequently requires that family members in the country of origin must wait until their sponsor in the United States files immigration paperwork, the immigration bureaucracy processes it, and their turn in the visa queue finally comes (which in some instances can take more than 10 years).[1] For unauthorized immigrants, border control initiatives have made it more expensive (and therefore more difficult) for families to enter the United States together. Often families remain separated until relatives in the United States earn enough money to pay for smugglers to facilitate the entry of family members. Family separation not only influences family dynamics and resources, but also means that family members will begin the acculturation process at different times. Sonia Nazario, in *Enrique's Journey* (2007), dramatically captured this dynamic of families striving for unification in her account of a young Honduran adolescent's effort to find his mother in the United States.

Family relationships and family obligations continue no matter how much distance there is between members. Social workers must develop an understanding of the serious responsibilities carried by the family members who are first to arrive, who continue to support those who remain "at home" in the country of origin. Adult members are obligated to send funds, clothing, medicine, and food—and these obligations often require them to work two or three jobs to make ends meet. This, in turn, contributes to children and adolescents spending a great deal of time at home without parental presence. Parents who find it difficult to negotiate the school system to support their children's education, largely because of language and cultural barriers, may, in fact, find it easier to work long hours; although it is necessary if they are to provide the necessities for family both here and "at home," they avoid encounters that are problematic and upsetting. For social workers, the challenge is to develop trusting relationships with immigrant families so that some of these hidden burdens can be shared and problem solving can take place.

Social work has been slow to recognize that many of our immigrant clients have limited English proficiency (LEP) and to develop strategies to ensure accurate and effective communication with those clients. Social work theorists from Perlman (1979) to Germain and Gitterman (1996) emphasize the centrality of relationship to social work practice—yet how can helping relationships be formed if social workers cannot communicate with their clients? This is not an obtuse, theoretical issue. People who have difficulty using English in their public interactions total more than 12 million persons, and they are among the most marginalized people social workers assist (Piedra, 2006). Curiously, the social work literature largely has been silent on service delivery to LEP clients, other than mentioning the need to have bilingual workers work with them. It appears that little thought has gone into how best to prepare bilingual social workers to use their language skills. Even less attention has been given to training monolingual-English social workers to work with interpreters. We know least of all how social service agencies assist LEP clients, the resources they devote to serving them, and what agency approaches are optimal.

IMMIGRANTS AND REFUGEES WITH SPECIAL NEEDS

Social workers are keenly aware of traditionally vulnerable populations, such as abused children and the homeless mentally ill, but are less knowledgeable about subpopulations of immigrants and refugees who do not readily seek social services even when they are in dire need. Survivors of torture, immigrant victims of domestic violence, and persons who have been trafficked are frequently hidden from view, partly because social workers do not know about them or do not ask the right questions to identify them, and partly because these persons fear that seeking assistance will put them at risk of further harm. However, trained social workers, who have learned about the special nature of the victimizations immigrants and refugees face, can begin to learn to ask the right questions; to probe carefully for cues that provide explanations and fill in the gaps; to reach out sensitively, carefully, and slowly while developing a trusting relationship. Social workers, who are trained in sensitive work with trauma survivors, whether in a health, mental health, employment assistance program, or school setting, can develop more appropriate care plans with the understanding that these clients will need more of their time, other resources, and a family- and community-based approach to resolving issues. This is indeed complex work, requiring specialized knowledge and skills. Specific training in work with survivors of torture is provided by some of the federally supported torture treatment centers across the country, and domestic violence work with immigrants occurs in most shelters. However, knowledge and skills in these areas are in need of considerable development, extension, and support. Finally, although the issues of human trafficking–and the lives of those it affects–are not new, the increased global movements of people demand social work's attention and learning.

Social workers also need to know that specific federal policy has recently been crafted to deal with certain immigrant populations that have experienced trauma and human rights violations. Over the past 20 years, the federal government has passed legislation to provide specific immigration status to certain groups of traumatized immigrants (refugees, asylees, battered immigrant women, and victims of trafficking) and has funded programs to address their trauma and facilitate their recovery (all the aforementioned plus survivors of torture). These federal policies are as important to immigrant practice as, for example, the Child Welfare Act of 1974 or ICWA are to child welfare.

SOCIAL WORK ADVOCACY

Because immigrants are considered outsiders by much of American society, they are easy scapegoats on whom to blame crime, terrorism, drugs, gangs, prison overcrowding, unemployment, welfare abuse, environmental degradation, and other social ills (Engstrom, 2006). Over the past decade, immigrants have seen their right to social protection eroded and their due process rights greatly curtailed. Immigrants have contested these assaults on their status and well-being, but have been largely unsuccessful in reversing anti-immigrant policies. It is here that the advocacy responsibility of social work acutely intersects with social justice and human rights issues for immigrants. The profession cannot sit by silently while immigrants get pushed even further to society's margins. Social workers involved in the well being of immigrants are in a perfect position to document the harm of anti-immigrant policies and to articulate the ways in which exclusion and xenophobia stigmatize and marginalize these populations.

At the turn of the 20th century, the energies of the best-known U.S. social worker, Jane Addams, focused on the needs of the immigrant poor and their communities. Now, a century later, it is vital that social workers reassume and reassert their role in the development, availability, and provision of services in immigrant communities, not necessarily as leaders, but in partnership with members of the community. When newcomers arrive, their natural inclination is to find others like themselves and their families, beginning with those who share their language and religious beliefs, and, above all, who can be trusted to help them re-establish their lives in this country. Enclaves begin to develop because most immigrants and refugees seek to live, work, and worship near each other based on ethnicity, clan membership, regional origin, and/or religious preferences, as well as availability and affordability of housing. Social workers should be working as a natural outgrowth of this process of community capacity-building. Immigrants and refugees come with a repertoire of survival abilities and resources that social workers can help tap once trust relationships have been established. Social workers need to return to these communities.

IMPLICATIONS FOR SOCIAL WORK CURRICULA

There are numerous considerations for change that would bring social workers back into immigrant communities. If we examine social work curricula with continued emphasis on clinical practice in field education, for example, we can see that innumerable academic requirements tend to restrict more creative opportunities for field learning, such as in ethnic communities where emerging organizations have neither MSWs or BSWs on staff. Less restrictive programs find means to pool supervision among several agencies to build capacity in newer community agencies. By adopting the need for reciprocal learning as a value, schools of social work and professional organizations could act in concert to bring members of new immigrant and refugee communities into the profession.

The implications of the preceding analysis are clear: Social work must develop specialization in immigrants and refugees just as it has in child, aging, and mental health. If social workers are to work competently with immigrants, their families, and their communities, schools of social work need to develop curricula that

- highlight an understanding of assimilation and acculturation;
- recognize the multitude of stresses and strains immigrant families experience;
- underscore the central role immigration status plays in shaping the life course of immigrants;
- emphasize the need to assist immigrants in dealing with the immigration, education, legal, health care, and social service bureaucracies;
- explore the Byzantine-like eligibility criteria for public welfare benefits;
- underscore the vulnerability of immigrants to private and public abuses of power;
- address the pre- and postmigration trauma and rehabilitation needs of certain immigrant groups;

- acknowledge the resiliency and resourcefulness of immigrants and craft interventions to build on those strengths.

This list is by no means exhaustive, but it does illustrate the complexity of immigrant practice and the need for social work to squarely address these issues.

NOTE

1. In some cases, family members may qualify for non-permanent immigration visas that allow them to reside temporarily in the United States until they obtain permanent immigration status. Many family members with valid visa applications, however, take the calculated risk of entering the United States illegally to be with their families. If apprehended by immigration authorities, they will be removed and barred from re-entering the country for 10 years.

REFERENCES

Engstrom, D. W. (2006). Outsiders and exclusion: Immigrants in the United States. In D. W. Engstrom & L. M. Piedra (Eds.), *Our diverse society: Race and ethnicity–Implications for 21st-century American society* (pp. 19-36). Washington, DC: NASW Press.

Fadiman, A. (1998). *The spirit catches you and you fall down: A Hmong child, her American doctors, and the collision of two cultures.* New York: Noonday Press.

Fix, M., & Zimmermann, W. (2001). All under one roof: Mixed-status families in an era of reform. *International Migration Review, 35*(2), 397–419.

Germain, C. B., & Gitterman, A. (1996). *The life model of social work practice: Advances in theory and practice.* New York: Columbia University Press.

Greeley, A. M. (2006). Why can't they be more like us? In D. W. Engstrom & L. M. Piedra (Eds.), *Our diverse society: Race and ethnicity–Implications for 21st-century American society* (pp. 3-8). Washington, DC: NASW Press.

Nazario, S. (2007). *Enrique's journey: The story of a boy's dangerous odyssey to reunite with his mother.* New York: Random House.

Perlman, H. H. (1979). *Relationship, the heart of helping people.* Chicago: University of Chicago Press.

Piedra, L. M. (2006). Revisiting the language question. In D. W. Engstrom & L. M. Piedra (Eds.), *Our diverse society: Race and ethnicity–Implications for 21st-century American society* (pp. 67-88). Washington, DC: NASW Press.

Diversity in Diversity: Changing the Paradigm

Rowena Fong

INTRODUCTION

As a child I felt tension between my first generation Chinese-speaking parents and myself, because we neither saw nor grasped the meaning of things the same way. Although we had never heard stilted terms like "intergenerational gap," "parent-child conflict" or "acculturation tensions," they aptly described my family. I always wondered how to explain to my parents, whose sole ambition for me was Harvard and a high paying job, that what I wanted to do was to be a social worker and teach about oppression, and how to practice social work in a way that was meaningful to others whose roots were in foreign soil, who had not grown up or lived long in America.

If my family situation were a fictitious case study in a social work class addressing culturally competent practice, what points would the instructor consider critical to the lesson? Certainly an instructor would hope to draw students' attention to the assessment stage and emphasize the need to do a thorough investigation of each family member. The instructor would urge students to determine how he or she described and experienced the tensions in the family. But would this assessment probe with any insight into what kind of Chinese family this was? What would the student social worker learn to ask about the family's Chinese cultural origins? How would the instructor explain the role of cultural values in the case study? Would anyone in the class wonder why education is so important to most Chinese families?

In assessing the case study situation, the perceptive social worker would note the clash between the parents' expectations and the child's reaction to those expectations. The social worker would anticipate gaps between the values of the parents and the child. The social worker might further clarify what appeared to be the presenting problem, and what could be the real problem in this family situation. Was the parent-child interaction actually cause for concern? Did the stress placed on the child's achievement seem entirely fair? While the scenario might seem a familiar parent-child conflict in any culture, what role does this family's ethnic community and the family's position in that larger milieu contribute to their tensions over education and work?

However talented or dedicated, no instructor could teach a social work student everything to look for surrounding the tensions in this Chinese family. Nor could the student learn everything to look for in other multicultural families. What the social work class instructor could hope to impart, however, are three things: a discernment of the complexity and differentness of their multicultural clients, an awareness of the family's legal status, and an ability to select culturally competent interventions that fit the multicultural client's unique needs.

DIVERSITY IN DIVERSITY

The instructor may first foster an appreciation of the complexity and differentness of the lives of their multicultural clients. Ethnic populations are seldom "all just alike." In fact, the diversity within the groups is often much more striking than any similarities. The Chinese population alone in the United States presents families with hundred year-old roots in the U.S., recent legal Chinese from the People's Republic of China with the one child policy, Chinese from Hong Kong, which had a British colonial government until transfer to Communist rule in 1997, and representatives of the Chinese Diaspora from Vietnam and Southeast Asia, East Africa, Latin America, and the Pacific Islands.

Within Asian American literature, it became important to distinguish Asians from Pacific Islanders. Among the Asian populations it was important to differentiate between East Asians (Chinese, Japanese, Filipino, Korean), Southeast Asians (Vietnamese, Cambodian, Laotian, Thai, and Burmese), and South Asians (Asian Indians, Pakistanis, Sri Lankans, and Bangladeshis). Among the Pacific Islanders were Hawaiians, Tongans, Samoans, Chamorros, Maoris, Fijians, and representatives of the many other islands scattered across the South Pacific. In areas with high rates of intermarriage, consciousness rose among racially mixed Hapa children and their families of their distinctiveness as individuals and as a group. Groups outside the Asia Pacific region have sub-groups and ethnic distinctions that are equally varied.

As in my own family, length of stay in the U.S. is commonly a critical feature, as well as age of arrival. As a child born in Boston, I saw matters quite differently from my parents who had migrated to the U.S. as adults. I adopted the Christian faith, and although I did go to superb schools, I wanted to pursue my own goals and ambitions in social work. Families longer established in the U.S., having made more adjustments to American culture, were likely to have fewer, less intense conflicts over cultural divisions.

Multicultural families from China or elsewhere also bring with them a socio-political background that bears on the job of the social worker. Families arriving from politically or economically unstable regions, who have suffered physical violence or large economic reversals, or who have experienced dramatic changes in their social status as a result of their move to the U.S. may all present different conditions to the social worker. Even after establishing themselves in the U.S., the family's affiliations with the ethnic community and the family's role in that community may add layers of complexity to their situation.

STATUS IN LAW

The social work instructor preparing social work students to work with multicultural clients may next convey some understanding of how the individual's ascribed status (usually legal) influences the social work intervention. Initially, social work tended to only note the difference between the American born ethnic groups and the foreign born. Among the immigrant population, however, it was important to pay attention to the differences between those who were immigrants and those who were refugees. Immigrants were people who were voluntarily leaving places of origin with the legal right to leave and enter to their home countries. Refugees were those persons who were being forced out of their homelands due to political turmoil with no option to return to their native counties. The circumstances that have compelled many to leave their homes frequently also result in higher than normal numbers of unaccompanied children among the refugees, and these also require special legal attention.

The most fundamental distinction of legal status, however, is that between those immigrants who were legal and those who were illegal or undocumented. The latter were individuals and families who voluntarily left their countries of origin and migrated to another country without legal documentation. These people are illegal and have a status that often does not allow them access to employment or social services in the United States.

The illegal families come seeking better lives and employment opportunities for the adults. Difficulties occur when the children of these families are caught in a mixed legal status. Some illegal children are barred from schools and services whereas their siblings who are born in the United States are U.S. citizens, which entitle them to services and education. Families of mixed legal status constantly grapple with the prospect of deportation and family separation, raising fears that complicate the task of the culturally competent social worker. Often the issues of "invisibility" and their "secret lives"–their lack of legal status and recognition–force them to become unknown (Fong & Earner, 2007, p. 418). Social workers have to respect these fears because they are real and constant in the lives of undocumented families. Yet, some of the undocumented families have mixed statuses when children of these families are born in the United States and have legal citizenships. How do culturally competent social workers serve members of the family who are illegal and a member who is legal? How does this legal diversity within the immigrant family get addressed?

I myself was born in the United States and grew up in an immigrant family whose legal status was never a problem, but our family's tensions were real due to racist attitudes and discriminatory practices against us. I can only imagine how much greater the tensions would have been if instead the scenario were I, the first born, was brought to America with my parents from China as an undocumented illegal child, and my brother was born here in American as a legal child. What kind of childhood could I have possibly had? My tensions with my parents would not have been about whether to go to Harvard or not, but instead it would be about whether I could attend school or not. If schooling and finding work were not options, then what was I suppose to do with my life? How could a social worker possibly help me feel better?

These are the questions social work students and professionals face today as they prepare for practice with immigrant and refugee children and families. Perhaps the familiar questions about the application of the National Association Code of Ethics need to be asked by the instructor about what the students in social work classes think about services offered to these mixed status families? Would the student have an ethical problem in offering social work services to a family that has an illegal member in it? Is it easier or harder for the student to offer services to an illegal immigrant or to a refugee whose religious faith differs from the dominant ones in the United States? These questions prevail.

Among the refugees who arrive in the United States are many who have transited through refugee camps before they can come to the United States. The most noteworthy piece of this history for the involved social worker is that refugee camps themselves, and the journeys to and from them, can be hazardous and brutal. Another group of people who are either immigrants or refugees, and who, in fact, may have come legally, are those deceived by the people who are supposed to help them come to the U.S. and fall victim to human trafficking. These victims, whether children or adults, can be exploited and enslaved as sex workers or slave laborers (Fong, Busch, Armour, Heffron, & Chanmugam, 2007). Can social work students and practitioners possibly understand the degree of trauma these children and families have experienced when their lives are so privileged by comparison, because they live in the United States and their attitudes of entitlement prevail? Can they really offer competent cultural practices without personal values and biases impeding their judgment and skills?

GOODNESS OF FIT

Finally, the social work instructor may strive to develop within students the conviction that assessments and interventions must be chosen to fit the multicultural client's unique needs. Those working with these clients must acquire and apply informed discernment. They need to better understand the social environments of the client, and how those environments influence the client's behavior. Understanding the client's historical, social, and political background permits the social worker to choose assessments and interventions that fit the client's needs. This task of understanding the background of an undocumented immigrant may be challenging for some social work students. While they may hear about the impoverished conditions of the country from which the undocumented family comes, and they may see in the news the war-torn neighborhoods and the starvation of children, yet the fact is that these people who are coming to settle into the United States do not have legal documents. They are outsiders, and the American government, newspapers, and newscasts are full of daily denunciations of this unwanted population "who are taking American jobs and are encroaching the welfare system" as they are so frequently portrayed.

Ethical dilemmas may arise when applying the goodness of fit test, in that the student social worker may have occasion to decide if the needs of the illegal client for food, clothing, shelter, and employment will fit with the social worker's goodness of heart and tendency towards social justice or instead fit with American societal pressure towards legalism and survival of the fittest. The fittest has usually been and continues to be defined as White, Anglo-Saxon, and Protestant.

The NASW Code of ethics and social work's core values emphasize social justice, dignity and worth of the person, integrity, and competence. Social work practitioners, educators, and students need to examine their practices to assure that illegal and undocumented immigrants or victims of human trafficking or persons of Muslim or non-Protestant faiths receive the kinds of assessments and interventions that meet their needs. However, in order to do this some continued honest introspection might still be needed. In 2001, the NASW Board of Directors approved the NASW Standards for Cultural Competence in Social Work Practice. Standard 2 on Self-Awareness states, "Social workers shall seek to develop an understanding of their own personal, cultural values and beliefs as one way of appreciating the importance of multicultural identities in the lives of people" (NASW, 2001, p. 1). Understanding, appreciating, and honoring of differences is absolutely necessary for culturally competent practice to occur.

CHANGING THE PARADIGM

In 2001, in the introductory chapter to a book I coedited with Sharlene Furuto on Culturally Competent Practice, I wrote,

> Multicultural social work addresses varied facets of culture, which include race, gender, age, sexual orientation, religion and so on. While multicultural social work includes these factors beyond ethnicity, the work remains to deepen the interracial, interblending of cultures found within the single ethnic group. . . . The knowledge of cultural competency that has been advocated in the past has focused on thinking and learning factual and descriptive knowledge about the client, with attributes presented as tangential to the functioning of the person or community. The value and belief system that comprise traditional and cultural norms need to be presented as central to the client's functioning. New paradigms and models need to be created to instill the practice of adopting the client's values as the norms. Social workers need to start with the ethnic environment of the client and use the larger, usually Euro-American norms only as they complement the client's ethnic reality (Fong & Furuto, 2001, p. 5).

The paradigm shift still awaits an awakening in culturally competent social work practice. The society in the United Sates is becoming increasingly multicultural with children and families from non-English speaking countries, particularly from Latin America and Asia. To continue to offer social work practice from solely a Western paradigm framework may be becoming obsolete (Fong, 2004). Standard 4 of the NASW Standards for Cultural Competence in Social Work Practice is entitled Cross-Cultural Skills and states, "Social workers shall use appropriate methodological approaches, skills, and techniques that reflect the role of culture in the helping process" (NASW, 2001, p. 1). Refugees from other countries had and continue to have ways of surviving and coping from stressors in their homelands. But as they enter the American social service delivery system, social work practitioners need to adjust the paradigm to prioritize and take the time in assessments to find out what are these existing strengths and coping skills of the foreign-born client. To seek commonalities of values and coping mechanisms should be the main goals of assessment and interventions rather than the practice of offering the convenient and conventional methods of treatment.

NASW Standards for Cultural Competent Practice summarizes the continued need for a paradigm shift by advocating,

> In the United States cultural diversity in social work has primarily been associated with race and ethnicity, but diversity is taking on a broader meaning to include the sociocultural experiences of people of different genders, social classes, religious and spiritual beliefs, sexual orientations, ages, and physical and mental abilities. . . . Therefore, cultural competence in social work practice implies a heightened consciousness of how clients experience their uniqueness and deal with differences and similarities within a larger social context (NASW, 2001, p. 2).

Legal status and political orientation need to be added to this list of diversity variables that intersect with race and ethnicity and embrace the sociocultural experiences of non-English speaking people coming to and living in the United States.

In summary, my main points are the diversity of our client population is very challenging, causing culturally competent practice to be multidimensional by including the variables of legal status and political orientation to be factored in the racial and ethnic backgrounds of clients. Knowing the sociocultural environments of a client is a must to understand his or her behaviors, whether the client is legal or illegal. Social work educators and practitioners need to know and understand the client's history and migration story to help fulfill the client's complex needs. The client's legal, political, as well as social and cultural factors, are important in the assessment and treatment planning stages of social work practice. There may be ethical dilemmas for social work students and educators about choosing how to handle children and families of mixed status backgrounds, because of potential clashes between personal and professional values. Finally, culturally competent practice needs to be taught and practiced in a different paradigm from the traditional Western framework, which may be becoming obsolete because of competing cultural values, non-comprehensive assessments, and culturally incompatible interventions.

REFERENCES

Fong, R. (Ed.). (2004). *Culturally competent practice with immigrant and refugee children and families*. New York: Guilford Press.

Fong, R., Busch, N., Armour, M., Heffron, L., & Chanmugam, A. (2007). Pathways to self-sufficiency: Successful entrepreneurship for refugees. *Journal of Ethnic & Cultural Diversity in Social Work*, Vol. 16, No. 1/2, 127-160.

Fong, R., & Earner, I. (2007). Multiple traumas of undocumented immigrants–Crisis enactment play therapy: Case of Ximena, Age 12. In Nancy Boyd Webb (Ed.), *Play therapy with children in crisis: Individual, group, and family treatment.* (pp. 408-425). New York: Guilford Press.

Fong, R., & Furuto, S. (Eds.). (2001). *Culturally competent practice: Skills, interventions, and evaluations*. Boston, MA: Allyn and Bacon Press.

National Association of Social Work. (2001). Standards for Cultural Competence in Social Work Practice. Washington, DC: Author.

Reflections on 30 Years of Advocacy, Thinking, and Writing About Elderly Latinos

Alejandro Garcia

INTRODUCTION

I have been writing about older Hispanics for over the past 30 years, and now I am one. Over that period of time, older Hispanics have changed as the larger society has changed, and I have changed. I do not believe that aging has provided me with any great wisdom about older

Latinos. If anything, it has challenged me with new questions about the aging process and about the social milieu within which we age. The intent of this essay is to reflect on the evolution of this group and my thinking on the issue.

In reflecting on my work over the years, I have found that things are not as simple as I once described them. When I first wrote about Mexican American elderly, I saw them as being rather homogeneous. I now recognize the complexity of the Latino elderly as their interactions with the larger society not only change them, but also change the larger society. To discuss a particular ethnic group without discussing its social context provides only an incomplete perspective of that particular group.

I remember that the first article I published 35 years ago was about working with Mexican American elderly, and I pointed out some of the cultural differences between this group and non-Hispanic White elderly. If I had to do that article at this time, I would have to consider a number of factors. The complexities of the various groups of Latino elderly require exploration: What is their country of origin? Are they recent immigrants or were they born in the United States? Were they urban or rural in their country of origin? What is their socioeconomic status? Where do they fit in the continuum of acculturation to American culture? All of these factors have implications for working with Latino elderly or for policy development that is responsive to their needs.

While most of my writing has been based on quantitative analyses, I would like to include some personal observations involving my own family, as its members have provided me with continuing insights into aging and Latinos in the United States. My mother, Josefina, died at age 92 in 2004, and my father, Arturo, died at age 87, seven years before my mother, in 1996. Both of my parents immigrated to the United States as rather young children during the Mexican Revolutionary War (1910-1920). All of their children were born in Texas.

I never knew either of my grandfathers, as they both died before I was born. I did know both of my grandmothers, who lived to see me grow to early adulthood. However, future generations of older Latinos will get to see children and grandchildren grow to adulthood, taking into consideration the increasing life expectancy of Latinos.

Our first language was Spanish, and I did not speak a word of English until I enrolled in public schools. My early socialization was that of a traditional, lower class, Mexican family, but the influence of public schools and higher education, as well as socialization outside of my Mexican barrio, took its toll on that socialization. In essence, this retrospective assessment of my work combines my own life experiences with my professional development.

THE LATINO FAMILY: A MORE COMPLEX UNDERSTANING

The Hierarchical Latino Family

Many Latinos grew up in a family that was hierarchical. The father was the head of the household, but the mother had the responsibilities for day-to-day operations of the home. Children were taught to treat adults with respect, especially their parents and grandparents. In addition, children were taught directly or by example that the family came first and the individual family member came second. The needs of the individual had to be subverted to the needs and wishes of the family. One may still find some of these behavioral characteristics in more traditional homes, but not in families that have had more exposure to socialization with the majority society in this country.

Generational Cultural Dissonance in the Changing Latino Family

As younger Latinos get socialized into the majority culture via the schools and peers, changes occur within generations of the family. The child may become exclusively English speaking, with his/her parents being bilingual, but grandparents being monolingual in Spanish, especially if they are immigrants from Mexico. But it is more than just language differences that separate generations within a family. Adaptation to a culture that emphasizes individualism versus collectivism, competition versus cooperation, and egalitarianism within the family versus a hierarchy may cause serious generation cultural dissonance within the family, as expectations regarding a number of matters may very greatly between generations.

In working with Latinos, a therapist will have to assess to what degree acculturation has occurred and the extent to which the family in question still maintains a strong, collective family orientation, or whether its members have become more independent, reflecting the values and practices of the majority society.

Fictive Kin and Informal Networks

One of the additional areas of study that I propose is the extent to which fictive kin continue to be part of the extended Latino family. To what extent do relations between *compadres* (parents and the godparents of a child) and between the godparent and godchild still exist? Traditionally, the parents selected close friends as godparents to baptize their children, and godparents were supposed to take care of the children should something happen to their parents. This *compadrazgo* was to cement a relationship between the various parties. In Mexico, one still hears people referring to each other as *compadre* and introducing these individuals to others by this status, rather than by name.

Another component of the extended family is *hijos de crianza*. This categorization, which literally means "children by rearing," applies to children who have been informally adopted by a family. They may or may not be blood relatives, but they become an integral part of the family.

The *barrio* or neighborhood has served as a source of support, particularly for monolingual and un-acculturated Latinos. As neighborhoods change and become more integrated, this will be a loss to the integrity of the *barrio* and to its function as a support system.

These traditional elements have been sources of mutual support and would continue to be a valuable asset as people age. The question is the extent to which these institutions will continue to be viable elements in the life of older Latinos.

Additional study should be carried out to determine whether older persons are increasingly using social service agencies or whether they are continuing to depend on the extended familial support system, the church, and their *barrio* (neighborhood).

Factors Influencing the Latino Family

The fact is that things have changed. In some ways, Latino elderly are doing much better economically, but, depending on their level of acculturation into American society, they may not better off otherwise. If the family has maintained some of the values of Latino culture, such as a collectivistic family that values the elderly, then the elderly person will be better off. However, if the elderly person still holds such values, but his adult children and grandchildren do not, then we can expect generational cultural dissonance to affect the relationship. In cases in which the elderly Latino is an immigrant who continues to main Spanish as his/her sole or primary language, this may form an additional gap between generations, as children and grandchildren may be more proficient in English or have English as their sole language of communication.

At this point in time, it appears that we are having a *d¾j' vu* experience when we see an increasing number of Latino grandparents taking primary care responsibility for their grandchildren. As a result of HIV/ AIDS, drug addiction, criminal behavior, and other factors, Latino grandparents have to assume responsibility for grandchildren. The collective orientation of the Latino family pushes this responsibility onto the grandparents, even though younger generations of the family may not have mutual perspectives regarding caring for older generations of their respective families.

CUENTOS *AND REMINISCENCES*

Latinos as Storytellers

I grew up in a world full of fables and fantasy. Latinos are recognized as great storytellers, and my family fit in well. As a child, I remember the world was full of storytellers. Older adults, as well as children, told *cuentos*, tales about ghosts and other apparitions, heroes, and gun fights. Once told, these tales took on a life of their own and were embellished to suit the occasion. Older persons were especially recognized for their abilities to tell these tales, and I remember being mesmerized by many of these tales about ghosts, Pancho Villa and the gold treasure that can be found somewhere in the state of Chihuahua, and the young woman who went to a dance without parental permission only to find out that she was dancing with the devil when she noticed he was dancing on his hooves, not his feet! These were more than fables, with many of them having a message about values imbedded within.

As we advance to a more technologically advanced society with children and young people preferring television, Ipods, and electronic games, I am concerned that we are losing this oral storytelling tradition and with it, the wisdom of our elders.

Reminiscences

Added to these *cuentos* were reminiscences about old days. My mother spoke about an aunt who followed her husband into battle with Pancho Villa's troops during the Mexican Revolutionary War. There were also stories about lining up at the *"relife"* (the relief distribution station) set up by the railroad tracks to distribute surplus food to hungry people during the Great Depression. One of my uncles also spoke about working the in the fields in South Texas during the Great Depression, but only being able to work half a day, because the other half day of work was reserved for Anglos (the non-Hispanic White workers).

My personal reminiscences include the *tamaladas* (tamale-making get-togethers) at Christmastime. While many people love to eat *tamales* (cornmeal dough rolled with shredded pork or other meat seasoned with a pepper sauce, wrapped in corn husks, and steamed), they do not know the extensive preparation that goes into making them. In my parents' home, my mother ruled the kitchen, but other female relatives would gather for this event. Men were definitely prevented from entering the kitchen, although as Mom grew older, she allowed me to help in the initial preparation of the meat filling and the corn dough. Some of the participants were better at chopping the meat or mixing the *nixtamal* (corn dough), while others specialized in soaking the corn husks or spreading the dough on the corn husks before another put in the filler and folded the corn husk before stacking it and placing it into what seemed like a mountain of tamales when I was a child. The uncooked tamales were then placed carefully in a circle in a rather large dish that resembled one of the tubs that we used to wash clothes. Hot water was placed over the tamales and then they were allowed to steam for what seemed liked an eternity for the children. All of us waited with great anticipation for the tamales to cook, and once the aroma of corn and spices permeated the house, we would start to compete for being first in line to get a hot *tamal*.

Canciones, Cuentos, Leyendas, and Dichos: Therapeutic and Philosophical Uses

Some therapists use "milestoning" to recapture positive memories that can balance present distressing circumstances or being stuck in negative memories. What were the milestones in a person's life–birthdays, deaths, deportation, weddings, quinceaneras (coming out celebrations for 15 year-old Latina girls), and year of immigration or naturalization? Persons can celebrate special occasions and survival and can give credit to themselves for their contributions to their families and society.

In a group the therapist could have theme reminiscing: perhaps around birthdays, celebration for el dia de los Santos or el dia de los muertos or de todos los santos, traditions in Mexico or in earlier days that may have been lost. For example, for el dia de los muertos, were there extensive preparations in building *arcos* in the house decorated with *cempasuchiles* (marigolds), which is the traditional flower for the dead, to honor dead relatives. Did the entire family go to the *camposanto* to clean up the grave of their dearly departed and to celebrate their memory on that day?

There can be group reminiscing: what was *la cocina* (kitchen) like in their youth? What was used for heat? Was it coal, gas, *brasas* (charcoal)? What were favorite dishes? *Tamales, chile verde, bunuelos* for New Year's? What was *"el dia del mercado"* (market day) like?

It would be wise for the therapist to know something about the history of Mexican Americans (or other Latino groups) in the United States and their migration. As in the case of my parents' cohort, knowledge of the Mexican Revolutionary War, 1910-1920, would be important. Elderly persons may have had relatives who fought with Pancho Villa or Emiliano Zapata. This period of unrest in Mexico may have also been the period for their family's migration to the United States.

The Great Depression is a time period of importance to many elderly Mexican Americans for a number of reasons. Not only was there tremendous despondency among this group in that period, but there was also concern for their immigration status. It was during this period that Carey McWilliams wrote about the thousands of persons of Mexican descent who, when they went to ask for public assistance, were repatriated to Mexico with their American-born children. McWilliams suggested that it was an economic decision: it would cost less to repatriate Mexican families than to support them on public assistance for one year. Abraham Hoffman (1974) suggested that there were over 400,000 persons of Mexican descent who were "repatriated" during this period, but the impact of this unethical, inappropriate and perhaps unconstitutional action may have affected many more Mexican Americans who remained in the United States.

The deportation of over 3.5 million undocumented aliens during Operation Wetback in the early 1950's may also be of import to elderly Mexican Americans. Older persons may recall drawing the blinds in their house as the Border Patrol vans passed through the streets of the barrio and being subjected to questions by immigration personnel on the streets, at work, and in the fields. What do you do when the *"la migra"* van comes by your neighborhood? As children, we learned that we were to go inside and pull down the shades until the van passed by. We also learned to carry our birth certificate with us at all times, in case we were stopped by *"la migra"* and asked to show our papers. This was not an infrequent event.

Racism is one of the issues that can be addressed through reminiscing. How did Latino elderly survive the ubiquitous racism that they faced? How were they able to maintain their pride, their integrity? How were they able to explain their physical differences to their children and support a positive perspective? Some elderly persons may do it through a *cuento* or folk tale. One *cuento* says that God created all of us in an oven. He left Mexicans in the oven just the right amount of time, and we came out a perfectly golden or bronze color. Other elderly persons may provide a quote for you: "*Si tu piel es morena, tienes suerte: el sol quiso estar cerca de ti.*" (If your skin is dark, you are lucky: the sun chose to be close to you.)

Reminiscence work with the elderly should not be limited to therapists. Families should also get involved in using reminiscence to promote intergenerational learning and respect. Encouraging the elderly to reminisce within the family will also support the traditional role of grandparents as providers of wisdom, moral guidance, traditions, and oral history.

My own work with Virginia Satir required that I do a family life chronology with my parents prior to beginning the training. I was going to carry out this task over the phone, but I had a sense that I'd better do it in person. In fact, when I sat with each of my parents out in their back yard, they both cried as they told me about their rather difficult childhood. I believe that such an exercise was mutually beneficial. I learned more about them then I had ever known in my life. I had a general sense about their experiences, but had not asked, and they had not shared these with me. I learned about their survival skills in spite of poverty and mistreatment and being taken out of school rather early in life in order to be treated like servants by other relatives. I believe that their sharing this information with me validated their experience and, essentially, their life, and made me appreciate them even more.

Dichos (Refranes)

Another way to elicit reminiscences is through sharing *dichos* or *refranes*. *Dichos* or *refranes* (proverbs or sayings) are popular guiding words that have existed for centuries in Latino cultures. They are lessons learned and words of wisdom that have guided generations through the ages with simple common phrases that combine wisdom with common sense. I remember that, on at least a couple of occasions, I addressed Latino elderly at conferences. So familiar was the audience with the *dichos* that I would provide the group with the first part of a *dicho,* and they would respond in unison with the second part of the saying. Most of the audience knew the sayings and had been repeating them and using them as behavioral guidelines throughout their lives.

One way to initiate reminiscences or validation for past accomplishments is to invite elderly Latinos to recall *dichos* or folk sayings common in the family.

In inviting elderly Latino clients or patients to recall *dichos*, the therapist may draw on this toward reminiscences or to expand on a family philosophical perspective. My father used to say *"El que al alva se levanta, tiene una hora mas de vida y en su trabajo adelanta."* (the equivalent of early to bed, early to rise. . . .) However, he quickly followed this up by countering this with *"No, no, no. . . . El que al alva se levanta, pierde de dormir un rato y cualquier bulto lo espanta"* (on the contrary, he who rises early loses sleep and is frightened by any dark shadow . . .).

Some of these sayings are simply common sense advice. For example, *"Al que le duele la muela, que se la saque."* (if you have a toothache, get it extracted) or more simply, if you believe that something is wrong, do something about it. The same applies to *"Perro que no sale no encuentra gueso."* (In other words, you need to work to get anything accomplished.)

Some are somewhat fatalistic and place one's situation in God's hands: *"A quien Dios quiera, le llena la casa de bienes"* (If God loves you, He will provide for you) or *"El hombre propone, Dios dispone."* (Man proposes, but God disposes) Other fatalistic perspectives include the following:

"El arbol que nace torcido, nunca se endereza. (You will never be able straighten a bent tree)

There are a number of dichos which provide advice. For example,

"El que no agarra consejo no llega a viejo." (He who does not accept advice will not live to old age)

"El que perdona a su enemigo a Dios tiene por amigo." (He who forgives his enemy will have God as a friend)

Or

"Guarda los centavos que los pesos llegaran." (Save your pennies; dollar bills will follow.)

"Haz bien y no mires a quien." (Do good deeds without first determining who the benefactor is.)

There is also is the following saying: *"Hijo eres, padre seras. Lo que con tu padre hicieres, contigo tus hijos haran."* In other words, you are someone's child now and you will be a parent in the future. The way you treat your parents now will be the way your children treat you in the future.

ADDITIONAL CONSIDERATIONS

Fatalismo

Do Latinos still believe in fatalism as extensively as I thought at the beginning of my academic career? I remember writing the oft repeated phrase among Latinos in response to some event: *"Asi lo quiso Dios."* (God willed it so.) I believe that such fatalism is still present, but that an analysis that examines Latinos according to socioeconomic status might yield a variety of responses, with upper class Latinos being considerably less fatalistic than lower class Latinos. My sense is that a lack of options tends to reflect fatalism, and that impoverishment tends to limit those options.

Better education has also resulted in enlightenment about the causes of poverty. Latinos are better able to examine structural causes of poverty, such as discrimination, rather than internalizing such causes and seeing poverty as individual deficiency.

English Language Fluency

Much has been written about limitations with English language fluency among the elderly Latinos, but not as much has been said about Spanish language fluency. We need to do more research on elderly Latinos and the degree to which they are fluent in either language. Due to low educational attainment levels, it is possible that they may be functionally illiterate in both languages, and it is important that we recognize this issue and find effective ways to communicate, such as personal visits, radio, and television, rather than through correspondence and pamphlets.

The fact is that a majority of older Latinos either prefer to speak Spanish or are monolingual in Spanish. Using interpreters to help in completing necessary forms may be acceptable, but for more complicated tasks, this may be a major challenge. If a social worker wants to do clinical work with Latino elderly, this may be difficult simply because of the verbal and nonverbal cues that need to be translated.

An additional issue is the question of who is used as an interpreter. We tend to be rather careless about this, sometimes using the most readily accessible person, rather than the most appropriate one. In our rush to get someone to translate for us, we sometimes forget about issues of confidentiality and respect for the client's privacy. One additional issue is the use of children in the home to provide translations. In using children to interpret for adults, a therapist has to keep in mind the appropriateness of discussing certain matters in front of the child and of the possibility of changing the power relationship between parent and child. In a hierarchical family like the Latino family, this may have important repercussions resulting in the adultification of the child and the diminishment of the adult's authority.

CONCLUSION

This has been a reminiscence exercise for me in recalling my work and my family. I have learned much from Latino elderly in my family and beyond. Latino elderly deserve to be able to live and celebrate this latter period of their lives in a way which generates respect and validation of their accomplishments. To not draw out their lifetime ability to survive in the midst of discrimination and poverty and to help them to validate their lives is, at minimum, a *"falta de respeto."*

Upon reflection, I want to thank all the major actors in my life, especially my parents, but other role models as well, for their contributions to my development. In doing so, I want to use an unpublished piece that I have used to thank older Latinos:

I believe that what has been lacking in the program today is an appropriate recognition of the senior citizens of the Hispanic community. We need to share our appreciation for we are deeply indebted to them. We need to celebrate *El Oro del Barrio*–the "Treasure in our barrio"–the senior citizens of the Hispanic community. I believe that the time has come to appreciate–not to denigrate–our senior citizens.

I believe that the time has come to tell the government that it needs to recognize and support our culture–not destroy it! It appears to me that the government does not appreciate–perhaps does not know–that the elderly in the Hispanic family are highly valued and have many responsibilities in our culture. For example, the government needs to know that the elderly in the Hispanic community are highly regarded for their wisdom. The elderly in the Hispanic community are highly respected for their knowledge of our history and our antecedents. The elderly in our community are respected because they have an important role in the socialization of our children, so that they can grow up with positive Hispanic values. The elderly in the Hispanic community are considered arbiters in the resolution of family problems. Whenever we have problems, to whom do we reach out? To our elderly relatives, of course.

Unfortunately, it appears to me that the government does not understand our culture; it does not understand our elderly. For example, the government reduces public assistance benefits for our senior citizens who live with other family members. It does not understand the value of the extended family in our culture. The government provides housing for the elderly, but it does not allow nephews or grandchildren to stay overnight. It does not understand the value of family members for our elderly.

Now is the time for change in government policies so that our culture is taken into consideration in the development of those policies. Our language and culture are not honored and recognized in many parts of this state and our country.

I believe that now is the time to show our appreciation for the treasure in our barrio–our Hispanic elderly. We have certain responsibilities toward our families and our elderly to help them survive in this world. We need to celebrate the accomplishments of our elderly in the Hispanic community.

I thank Latino elderly for their wisdom, their graciousness, their character, and their love.

REFERENCES

Hoffman, A. (1974). Unwanted Mexican Americans in the Great Depression: Repatriation pressures, 1929-39. Tucson: University of Arizona Press.

McWilliams, C. (March 1933). Getting rid of the Mexicans. *The American Mercury.*

Zuniga, M. E. (Undated). Mexican Americans and Reminiscence: Interventions Available: http://www.haworthpress.com/store/E-Text/View_EText.asp?sid=T6CG73AH7GE89N8F7FEEGRFD2U7EDE2A&a=3&s=J083&v=14&i=3%2F4&fn= J083V14N03_05

Latino Cultural Assets and Substance Abuse Services: Opportunity Knocks

Melvin Delgado
Lisa de Saxe Zerden

INTRODUCTION

The Latino community has certainly received considerable public recognition as the result of the debates concerning unauthorized entrance into the United States. However, within social work and human service circles, this community has a long history of recognition and has played an important role in pushing forth an intervention and research agenda embracing cultural competence (Crunkilton, Paz, & Boyle, 2005; Delgado, 2007). Nevertheless, there is much more progress that must be made in all fields of practice, with substance abuse being no exception (Delgado, 2005a). How the field of substance abuse responds to the challenges of better understanding and serving the needs of Latinos, an increasingly diverse group, will dictate the relevance of the field for this community in the present and in the near future.

This article explores the potential for utilizing Latino cultural assets for research and programming of substance abuse services, and identifies some of the reasons why these assets have generally been untapped by the field of substance abuse, and what can be done this decade to rectify this situation. A case illustration of Latino Pentecostal churches and alcohol, tobacco, and other drug abuse will be highlighted to illustrate how cultural assets must be taken into account when working within the field of substance abuse. The complexities of identifying and mobilizing indigenous assets within marginalized urban communities in the United States are bound to present challenges. Nevertheless, the potential rewards of success far outweigh these challenges regarding time and effort.

DEMOGRAPHICS

The subject of demographics plays an influential role within the field of substance abuse, as it does in other fields, particularly when regarding the Latino community in the United States (Miranda, 2005). An understanding of demographics provides important direction for where and how to conceptualize service delivery. However, when applying demographics to Latinos, it is necessary to take into account the multi-subgroups that can be found within this community. The issue of undocumented status, for example, is no longer just a regional factor to take into account, since all regions of the country have or are currently experiencing an upsurge in representation (Delgado, Jones, & Rohani, 2005). Geographical areas with high concentrations of undocumented residents present social workers with different challenges when compared to areas with minimal representation of undocumented residents.

Latinos numbered almost 42 million in 2005, or 14.5% of the total population (Pew Hispanic Center, 2006), and they are projected to encompass 25% of the nation's population by 2050 (U.S. Census Bureau, 2005), representing an increase of 49% from 2000 (Delgado, 2007). The

Latino community is quite diverse in backgrounds and consists of 29 different subgroups, with Mexicans (66%), Puerto Ricans (10%), and Dominicans, Cubans and Salvadorans (3%, respectively) representing the largest Latino groups in the United States (U.S. Census Bureau, 2005).

SUBSTANCE ABUSE

The field of substance abuse has started to pay close attention to the role and consequences of alcohol and other drug abuse in the Latino community (De La Rosa, Holleran, & Straussman, 2005). Part of this attention has been the direct result of the increased number of Latinos residing in the United States and the nature of acculturation, dispersal, and settlement patterns. The concentration of Latinos within the nation's urban areas, particularly in large cities with increased media outlets such as Chicago, Miami, Los Angeles, and New York, for example, has served to further highlight how Latinos are changing the political, social, and economic landscape of the nation. Although the problem of substance abuse among Latinos is well acknowledged by both professionals and the community, there are tremendous unmet needs for alcoholism and other substance abuse treatment services (Wells, Klap, Koike, & Sherbourne, 2001).

CULTURAL ASSET PARADIGM

The field of substance abuse has embraced the importance of culture in influencing health beliefs, behaviors, and help-seeking patterns. This embrace, as a result, plays an influential role in helping to shape substance abuse interventions at the primary, secondary, and tertiary levels (Hecht & Krieger, 2006). Culture fulfills a variety of important functions, not least of which is helping individuals socially navigate their way through society. Consequently, there is no aspect or arena of substance abuse that does not benefit from inclusion of Latino cultural assets as a means of increasing cultural relevance and competency. However, any effort to identify, include, or mobilize cultural assets is not without thorny conceptual and methodological research challenges, such as the role of acculturation in altering cultural assets. Culture is never a static construct, and is meant to be dynamic to accommodate local circumstances to help ensure group survival.

A cultural assets paradigm represents a significant shift in how the field of human services view Latinos and other marginalized groups in society. The prevailing perspective on these groups can be easily characterized as "deficit-driven" with an almost exclusive emphasis on identifying problems and inabilities to cope in this society. A cultural asset paradigm can be defined as: " . . . a construct that represents the beliefs, traditions, principles, knowledge, and skills that effectively help people, particularly those who are marginalized economically and socially by a society, to persevere and succeed in spite of immense odds against them" (Delgado, 2007, p. 20). In the case of Latinos in the United States, cultural assets represent "capital" that can be manifested in service to the community in addressing needs related to substance abuse.

The emergence of this construct in nontraditional settings typifies how cultural assets can be conceptualized and utilized in substance abuse service provision. Nontraditional settings can be defined as places in a community where residents go to purchase a product or service or go for recreation. In the process of doing so, they receive a wide range of what can be considered social services (Delgado, 1998). Each community will have their own version of nontraditional settings, such as beauty parlors, barbershops, grocery stores, and houses-of-worship, for example. These cultural resources coexist with conventional formal resources, and do so in parallel fashion.

Delgado and Rosati (2005), for example, researched the role of Latino Pentecostal churches in providing substance abuse services to their congregation in a New England city and found that many of these institutions were providing a wide range of services including counseling, support groups, and in some cases, detoxification. However, none of these Pentecostal churches reported any form of collaboration involving formal substance abuse services. Churches with ministers in recovery were more likely to offer substance abuse services than those headed by ministers without substance abuse histories. This cultural asset, however, existed in parallel fashion with formal services without the benefit of interacting with or receiving any form of support for a population group that was generally underserved. Unfortunately, a potential opportunity for the field of substance abuse to collaborate with this community's cultural asset was overlooked.

Delgado and Rosati (2005) identified seven ways that Pentecostal churches can play an important role in the field of substance abuse: (1) *training*: involving ministers in training substance abuse staff on how religious beliefs have been incorporated into service delivery; (2) *prevention*: distribution of materials and videos highlighting this cultural asset; (3) *resource utilization*: collaborative ventures involving Pentecostal churches; (4) *promoting alternatives through community education*: co-sponsorship of community education workshops on substance abuse; (5) *enhancing social competence*: co-leadership of workshops focused on congregational membership; (6) *policy development*: involvement of church leadership in advocating policy makers for funding of Latino-focused services; and (7) *guiding principles*: incorporation into the field of substance abuse many of the guiding cultural asset principles used in service delivery by Pentecostal congregations.

ACCULTURATION

Within social work practice, the "person in environment" perspective is a seminal framework practitioners employ to more fully appreciate the lives and contexts in which people live. Given this importance, how individuals and groups fit within their environment has been a crucial factor in understanding how acculturation affects one's pattern of behavior, mores and beliefs (Chun, Organista, & Marín, 2002). Acculturation, the process which entails the social and psychological exchanges that take place when there is contact and interaction between individuals from different cultures (Clark & Hofsess, 1998), has consistently been found to be positively associated with Latino substance abuse (Gil, Wagner, & Vega, 2000; Ortega, Rosenheck, Algería, & Desai, 2000). Yet, within the field, as with any phenomenon influencing Latino health, the role of acculturation requires the consideration of various cultural attributes, language proficiency, nativity, and migration and immigration patterns among other characteristics that differ within Latino sub-groups. Furthermore, existing literature focusing on substance use and the acculturation processes has measured acculturation in varying ways. This has resulted in discrepant findings, making it difficult for providers to discern best practices for substance abuse treatment and services.

Various studies have used different measures of acculturation, making comparison studies quite difficult (Chun et al., 2002). Although an array of acculturation measures have been designed to quantify the behaviors, values and attitudes of the Latino population, a major criticism within acculturation literature is the lack of clear definitions and conceptualization of acculturation markers (Hunt, Schneider, & Comer, 2004). Another criticism of existing acculturation measures is their inability to capture the developmental processes that may vary depending on when in life the person flows between cultures. This is particularly salient within substance abuse as different life stages and stressors may contribute to different patterns of use and treatment utilization throughout the life course. Additionally, an analysis of acculturation measurements has exposed a dearth of scales and definitions specific to substance using populations. Recommendations to improve existing scales include more uniform proxy measures of the acculturation process and the improvement in the operationalization of such factors (Cabassa, 2003). Most importantly, the context in which populations experience acculturation needs to be considered, especially through the lens of substance use, mental health, and viable treatment options.

The study of acculturation is necessary as "it represents critical socio-cultural and identifying characteristics of Latino populations with important implications for research and services" that can be tailored specifically towards Latino substance using populations and their families (Yamada, Valle, Barrio, & Jeste, 2006, p. 520). As such, the applicability of acculturation needs to be critically examined in order to attend to the challenges and experiences of this population.

CONCLUSION

The utilization of Pentecostal churches in substance abuse research, training, and programming, is but one example of how Latino cultural assets can be tapped by the field. Latino cultural assets remain largely unrecognized and as a result, untapped. The role and importance of culture in helping to identify and mobilize indigenous resources is well understood in the profession of social work and the field of substance abuse.

The need for the profession and the field to be creative in better identifying and mobilizing cultural assets, however, has not progressed as far as needed and must continue to make significant strides in the decades ahead. Failure of the field to recognize indigenous cultural assets will result in a field that loses its relevance for a population group that will continue to increase numerically in the next forty years.

REFERENCES

Cabassa, L. J. (2003). Measuring acculturation: Where we are and where we need to go. *Hispanic Journal of Behavioral Sciences, 25*(2), 127-146.

Chun, K. M., Organista, P. B., & Marín, G. (Ed.). (2002). *Acculturation: Advances in theory, measurement, and applied research.* Washington, DC: American Psychological Association.

Clark, L., & Hofsess, C. L. (1998). Acculturation. In S. Loue (Ed.), *Handbook of immigrant health* (pp. 37-60). New York: Plenum Press.

Crunkilton, D., Paz, J. J., & Boyle, D. P. (2005). Culturally competent intervention with families of Latino youth at risk for drug abuse. In M. De La Rosa, L. K. Holleran, & S. L. A. Straussman (Eds.), *Substance abusing Latinos: Current research on epidemiology, prevention, and treatment* (pp. 113-132). New York: Haworth Press.

De La Rosa, M., Holleran, L. K., & Straussman, S. L. A. (Eds.). (2005). *Substance abusing Latinos: Current research on epidemiology, prevention, and treatment.* New York: Haworth Press.

Delgado, M. (2007). *Social work practice with Latinos: A cultural assets paradigm.* New York: Oxford University Press.

Delgado, M. (Ed.). (2005). *Latinos and alcohol use/abuse revisited: Advances and challenges for prevention and treatment programs.* New York: Haworth Press.

Delgado, M. (1998). *Social work practice in nontraditional urban settings.* New York: Oxford University Press.

Delgado, M., & Rosati, M. (2005). Pentecostal religion, asset assessment and alcohol and other drug abuse: A case study of a Puerto Rican community In Massachusetts. In M. Delgado (Ed.). (2005). *Latinos and alcohol use/abuse revisited: Advances and challenges for prevention and treatment programs* (pp. 185-203). New York: Haworth Press.

Delgado, M., Jones, K., & Rohani, M. (2005). *Social work practice with refugee and immigrant youth in the United States.* Boston: Allyn & Bacon.

Gil, A. G., Wagner, E. F., & Vega, W. A. (2000). Acculturation, familismo, and alcohol use among Latino adolescent males: Longitudinal relations. *Journal of Community Psychology, 28,* 443-458.

Hecht, M. L., & Krieger, J. L. R. (2006). The principle of cultural grounding based substance abuse prevention. *Journal of Language and Social Psychology, 25,* 301-319.

Hunt, L., Schneider, S., & Comer, B. (2004). Should "acculturation" be a variable in health research? A critical review of research on US Hispanics. *Social Science & Medicine, 59,* 973-986.

Miranda, C. (2005). Brief overview of Latino demographics in the twenty-first century: Implications for alcohol-related services. In M. Delgado (Ed.), *Latinos and alcohol use/abuse revisited: Advances and challenges for prevention and treatment programs* (pp. 9-27). New York: Haworth Press.

Ortega, A. N., Rosenheck, R, Alegría, M., & Desai, R. A. (2000). Acculturation and the lifetime risk of psychiatric and substance use disorders among Hispanics. *Journal of Nervous and Mental Disorders, 188,* 728-735.

Pew Hispanic Center. (2006). *Hispanics at mid-decade.* Washington, DC: Author.

United States Census Bureau (2005). *Projected population of the United Stated, by race and Hispanic Origin: 2000-2050.* Retrieved November 21 2006, 2006, from http://www.census.gov/ipc/www/usinteriorimproj/natprojtab01a.pdf

Wells, K., Klap, R., Koike, A., & Sherbourne, C. (2001). Ethnic disparities in unmet need for alcoholism, drug abuse and mental health care. *American Journal of Psychiatry, 158*, 2027-2032,

Yamada, A. M., Valle, R., Barrio, C., & Jeste, D. (2006). Selecting an acculturation measure for use with Latino older adults. *Research on Aging, 28*(5), 519-561.

REFLECTIONS ON TEACHING ABOUT DIVERSE POPULATIONS

Reflections on Introducing Students to Multicultural Populations and Diversity Content

Diane de Anda

INTRODUCTION

There is something both daunting and exciting about teaching a course whose underlying aim, even if not explicitly acknowledged, is to significantly change the students' views of themselves, the world around them (particularly the interpersonal world), and their relation to it. All teachers who believe in the importance of their subject matter, of course, hope that the knowledge they are imparting is transformative on some level. However, this is the primary mission of introductory courses focused on multicultural populations and diversity content, particularly in social work education programs. Such courses aim to help broaden the student's awareness of the diversity of perspectives, values, assumptions and the behavior that flows from these and, in turn, to become more aware of oneself in all these regards with the further objective of examining oneself and societal structures in relation to these "others."

I have had the fortune of many years of teaching and developing curricula in this role and at many levels, from junior high school to undergraduate and MSW courses at UCLA and even a doctoral colloquium focused on imparting the art and science of teaching such courses. In my early twenties, I was selected along with 13 other history teachers in the Los Angeles Unified School District to create and teach a new and very controversial course on the history of multicultural populations in the United States. We were all ingenues and, being the late 1960's, little material existed, especially for this grade level, but we took up the task with the enthusiasm and tenacity born of the era of the Civil Rights Movement.

The undergraduate courses have all been electives, with most students entering with motivation, or at least curiosity, to learn about culturally different others, and none suspecting that the course would also require them to also learn about themselves. As I have gone around the room and had students share why they have elected to take the course, there have also been the forthright few who report it was the only course that fit into their schedules; they suspect the least regarding the process that will occur over the course of the quarter. (For a detailed description of the process and content of the course, see de Anda, in press.)

For a decade, I have team taught the Cross-Cultural Awareness course, the required course in the second quarter of the MSW program that attempts to provide a comprehensive introduction to diverse populations and issues related to diversity at the micro and macro levels, all in the space of four hours per week over ten weeks. The course is designed to offer both breadth and intensity to build knowledge and create a transformative experience. (For readings on teaching as a transformative experience, refer to Lee & Greene, 2003 and Mesirow & Associates, 2000.)

The doctoral colloquium required not only an examination of my own teaching experiences to distill the structure and content for anxious doctoral students about to enter the job market in this teaching role, but to simultaneously model the methods and teacher characteristics I was describing.

For this article, I have attempted to identify the factors I feel have facilitated the learning process in these varied teaching experiences and some of the pitfalls I have also noted along the way. These are not presented as findings based on quantitative, empirical data, as has been the case in most of my published articles over the years, but, rather, as reflections based on observations of patterns over a number of years in a variety of teaching settings and structures and with a very diverse body of students.

THE TEACHER

My experiences and observations teaching alone or as a member of teaching teams who examined the process as well as the content of their courses each year, have led me to conclude that there are both teacher characteristics and behaviors that facilitate learning in courses on diversity. This is not to say that individuals who do not possess these characteristics cannot or should not teach these courses, but that achieving the course objectives may be more challenging in those circumstances.

Please note that I have purposefully chosen the word "teacher" rather than "instructor." An instructor, in my opinion, attempts to convey subject matter; they, quite simply, "instruct." A teacher, on the other hand, also "instructs," but with an aim toward the individual's growth not only in knowledge, but the integration of this knowledge in a way that furthers development of the whole person.

There has been an ongoing debate regarding whether a cross-cultural/multicultural course should (perhaps could) only be taught by persons of color. Some schools have taken a team teaching approach, employing individuals from a broad spectrum of ethnic/cultural groups in a co-teaching role. Without skirting the debate, my observations of the teacher's impact on the students has led me to conclude that what is critical is that the teacher be bicultural. By this I mean that the teacher must have had the experience of functioning in more than one "cultural world," that there must be some disparities between the two (this "other" cultural world and the mainstream culture), that this must have occurred during the person's formative years, and that the person has spent time reflecting upon how this bicultural existence has shaped who he or she is in various obvious and more subtle and covert ways. This experience is most common for people of color, and the four components described above are more readily recognized in their life histories and situations. However, I use the term "cultural world" in a very broad sense, that could include others as well. Some of the White students in my courses have provided vivid examples, from having been raised in a "biker culture," strict Jehovah Witness culture that made clear separation between their world and those who were not of their faith, or in a family whose lives were embedded in the culture of the Salvation Army. Despite fitting more easily by appearance into the majority White culture and its institutions than persons of color, these individuals experienced being an "outsider" and a "differentness" in their view of self at a profound level, as well as differential treatment from others who did not share their unique cultures. The same is true for White individuals who grew up with their identity also tied to an ethnic heritage that had clear values, norms, and perspectives that did not parallel the mainstream. This does not include individuals whose connection to their ethnic heritage is primarily symbolic, who roll out the ethnic trappings on special occasions and put away any ethnic identification or identity once the boxes of artifacts are put back in the cupboard or to those whose ethnic identification and connection are evident only behind the closed doors of family gatherings. For this latter group, closeting this part of self protects them from the experience of being treated as "other" in the mainstream culture. The person who has, for the most part, experienced privilege, no matter how well examined, based upon his/her majority status and has not had the experience of being "other" in some *significant* and *formative* way is not well-suited to communicate the cross-cultural experience.

The teacher needs to be willing and able to relinquish any authoritarian, and sometimes even authoritative, role. The learning in a cross-cultural class cannot be all top-down, imported from the professor. It must be lateral as well, with students sharing their own backgrounds, their new learnings about other cultural groups, the content and their feelings regarding field experiences and assignments. Students may at times fill in important information and examples to complement the content offered by the teacher. The teacher must be practiced in facilitating these contributions, as no one person can be expected to have expertise with regard to the growing number of diverse populations in the country. Student assistance, particularly from individuals who are members of the cultural group being addressed, should be welcomed and encouraged without the teacher feeling or conveying a sense of being threatened or embarrassed. The teacher must also beware of a pitfall, that of generalizing from the particular, which students in their inexperience may inadvertently do. The teacher must be aware of information that is idiosyncratic and sensitively make this distinction. Finally, the teacher also needs to be able to take the information provided by the students and connect it to the course readings and field experiences, and not expect students to do so on their own, at least initially.

The teacher needs to be able to create an atmosphere of safety and security in the classroom that will encourage students to share and question openly without the fear of being viewed or labeled negatively, especially by their peers. This involves risk. Because the teacher should never ask students to do something he/she would not be willing to do himself/herself, and because modeling is a very effective teaching method, the teacher must risk, in most cases by appropriate self-disclosure. Others (Garcia & Van Soest, 2000) have also identified the value of the teachers sharing their life histories, particularly with regard to examples of oppression. In my own teaching, I have found that it is important to share brief examples across the gamut of emotions and experiences, including humor, not just those of suffering and pathos. It is important that they be directly tied to specific content that is being covered at the time, that they be brief so that an inordinate amount of focus is not on the professor, and that this is immediately followed by asking if others in the class have similar experiences to share from other cultural groups, which facilitates the recognition of commonalities along with differences. The disclosure and sharing can be general and brief or complex and emotionally laden. For example, in discussing bicultural socialization (de Anda, 1984), I usually include the effect of having words in a person's culture of origin that have no English translation and give, as an example, a Spanish word from my own culture, *"asco,"* which I vividly describe as a revulsion so extreme as to cause a person to feel nausea. I immediately ask for examples from the students, who respond enthusiastically, sharing words from a variety of languages and cultures, the interest of their peers reinforcing this small risk. At other times in the course, I have shared the fear I felt as the first person in my family to enter college and one of only five or so Latinas in the entire student body. This modeling allowed, for example, a Cambodian student to share that he is known in his community as "the one who got out," the only one of his peers to not only go to college, but complete high school and not end up a victim of violence and/or drug abuse.

The teacher needs to be able to employ a strengths perspectives with regard to the various populations discussed in the class. Part of this comes with accurately conveying the historical and cultural context as well as the institutional and societal factors that impinge upon the various groups. But most important is the ability to identify the ways the culture contributes positively to the development and welfare of individuals and the group as a whole, particularly from the perspective of the values of the culture. One cannot assume that this is a given in the students' educational experience. Students from various ethnic/cultural groups (e.g., Mexican, Filpino, Vietnamese, Korean) have written notes or spoken to me privately offering appreciation for the first time they ever heard anyone in a university course talk about their cultural group in a positive manner.

Furthermore, the strengths perspective needs to be applied to the students in the class as well, helping them realize they have important knowledge to share rather than focusing on the breadth of their knowledge deficits with regard to diverse populations, which can immobilize students, particularly White students who sometimes begin the course feeling they have "no culture" compared to the persons of color in the class, who have examples to share with the class.

The teacher must feel and be able to communicate and engender enthusiasm. The students' degree of motivation will vary significantly when they enter the class, especially if it is a required course and also if the content appears somewhat threatening. The teacher needs to convey the sense that they are embarking upon an adventure, that this exploration will take them to new and fascinating worlds. The message must be communicated with affect, and this must be the case each time the class meets. The course requires talking about values and feelings of various groups under a great variety of circumstances; this cannot be done without expressing emotion as well. The instructor needs to model the expression of emotion as a valid component of the learning processes and as integrated with the cognitive components. This allows teaching to become a holistic process.

Finally, the teacher must listen to the students' discomfort and not just write it off as resistance. Students begin at different places and develop at different rates. It is important to explore the sources of discomfort and identify anything in the teaching approach or pace that might be contributing in a negative way. It is also important to recognize that some discomfort may be a natural component of the process, and that it just needs to be monitored and support provided to make sure that it does not become counterproductive.

THE STUDENTS

I am convinced that one cannot teach about diversity unless the class is composed of ethnically/culturally diverse students, at least to some degree. I have observed the remarkable learning that has taken place in my undergraduate classes with the greatest diversity, including students whose backgrounds are African American, American Indian, Armenian, Asian Indian, Belisian, Cambodian, Chinese, Czechoslovakian (from the Czech Republic), Egyptian, Filipino, Iranian, Japanese, Jewish, Korean, Latino (Mexican American, Central American, Puerto Rican), Syrian, Thai, Vietnamese and more; Los Angeles presents such opportunities. The diversity of students in the MSW program has not been as extensive, but has also contributed significantly to the learning experience and environment in both the large lecture and small group settings. Readings, guest speakers no matter how dynamic, and videos cannot equal the effect of these diverse peers listening to, discussing, and interacting with each other, often for the first time with others from these diverse cultures.

Having chaired or been a member of MSW admissions committees for more than 25 years, I have noted the general agreement that the ideal student body would be ethnically/culturally diverse with these individuals having experience across diverse populations. However, in both the undergraduate program and the MSW program, even though there may be a diverse group of students to a greater or lesser extent, the experience with diversity of these students may be very limited. I was surprised by the number of students in such a diverse metropolis who had never ventured beyond social circles which were culturally homogeneous, and even some who had not ventured beyond the confines of their geographically familiar community. The interaction with their peers provided a safe and supportive first step and a chance to go beyond the classroom and establish relationships, certainly less threatening for the MSW students than their culturally different clients. I have observed students from different Asian populations (Chinese, Japanese, Korean) approach each other for the first time to explore their commonalities and differences; a Latina take her first foray outside of her East L.A. Latino community secure in the encouragement and protection of her new multicultural peers; an African American student confess to the members of her discussion group that this was the first time she felt she could trust anyone outside of other African Americans to share her feelings about her cultural experience as manifested in her extended family; a White student find comfort and support from a Latino ex-homeboy after feeling devastated by comments of a guest speaker that she felt were an affront to her lesbian identity. The absence of diversity in the student body is not only a missed opportunity for important learning to occur; it also contradicts the basic premise of the course, the importance of diversity.

For MSW students, diversity in terms of age and experience is also critical, particularly with a growing trend of accepting students directly or one or two years out of undergraduate education. What is important is not just the broader range of experiences to share, but the opportunity for students to have their peers share personal experiences that illustrate how historical and changing societal contexts impact the populations and issues of concern in the course over time. For micro students, in particular, establishing relationships across age groups helps work against the tendency to over-identify with clients from one's age cohort, particularly counter-productive in family treatment.

Students must be willing to risk, a complement to the teacher's ability to create and maintain a safe learning environment. Risk in this case means sharing of self, one's background, one's learning and new insights (particularly those gleaned from field assignments), one's concerns and emotional responses to the material, one's peers, and/or one's experiences in the field. Risk is very individual, different in degree, and also reinforced or sanctioned differently in a person's family and culture. The instructor and peers need to be sensitive to this, and patient. It is my experience that even the most reticent student is ready to risk by the end of the course. Fortunately, there is always a critical core of students who pave the way and model for others, the first to risk and prove to their fellow students that it can be a safe and positive experience. It is crucial to insure that this is, in fact, a positive experience for the student and in the eyes of their peers; confrontation or lukewarm reception will encourage only those who enjoy adversarial interactions to risk. Most of the students will play it safe.

THE STRUCTURE

The courses I have taught have employed various structures, some by choice, some by the demands of the curriculum or the number of students who elected to take the course. These have included at the MSW level, seminars with 20 to 25 students, a large lecture format (100 students) followed immediately with smaller (20 to 22 students) discussion groups, and, at the undergraduate level, a lecture/discussion format with class size varying from 35 to 70 students. There are benefits and pitfalls in all of these forms, but the critical element which determines their success is, I believe, insuring a degree of intimacy.

Oddly enough, it was the seminar structure that was the least conducive to developing a sense of intimacy in the group. This was probably the case because covering all the course content left only limited time for group processing, and most of this was conducted as group exercises directly tied to the material for the day rather than out of the experiences of the members of the class.

Switching to the combined format of large lecture followed by small discussion groups (and doubling the class hours from two to four per week) allowed the content that was the focus of the day to be presented by those with the greatest expertise to all the students at one time, but also made it possible to deal with the often controversial and emotionally laden content in the safe environment of a small cadre of students with whom relationships had been built. Although about the same size as the previous seminar groups, these groups differed in that the focus was more on processing the content of the readings and the lecture on a more concrete and personal level, and addressing the experiences of individuals in the group in their personal and professional development. The groups were marked by significant intensity and intimacy built over time, which became privy to professional dilemmas, personal disclosure (including sexual orientation, histories of abuse, and intergenerational effects of discrimination and the immigration experience), and a strong supportive group culture. The evaluations at the end of the course each year (across all four groups facilitated by different faculty members), the department's yearly survey, and the testimonies of numerous second year students in their final oral comprehensive at the end of their final year in the program, all report the transformative effects of the course in this particular format, particularly the effect of the small group experience.

There are a few concerns and dilemmas I have noted with regard to the large lecture structure, particularly one which employs guest lecturers as well as a team of faculty members. Student learning is impeded in a cross-cultural awareness course if they are allowed to become passive. "Lectures" must be interactive to some extent, even in a large setting and must call for the students to bring their own experiences, questions, and dilemmas to the content at hand. Guest speakers share their particular area of expertise with the group, but do not necessarily tie it directly to the course content or materials. A decision needs to be made as to whether it is more effective for the faculty facilitators to use the small groups to make these connections or provide some structure ahead of time for the guest speakers. Finally, there is the paradox posed by the dynamic guest speaker. Charismatic and controversial guest speakers generate enthusiasm for the content and often a readiness to discuss the impact in the small group sessions that follow. However, it is important that style and charisma not overshadow or become more valued by the students than the learning process and their personal and professional development. I became aware of this curious situation when a student standing in a long line to have a her moment with the guest speaker after his presentation remarked about the course lectures, "It's like the rock stars of social work!"

THOUGHTS ON CONTENT AND METHOD

This will not be an attempt to provide an outline or summary of all the content that needs to be included in designing an effective course on multicultural populations and related issues. That has been done ably over the years by a number of well-respected experts in this area, including Devore and Schlesinger (1981-1999), Green (1982-1999), and Lum (1999 & 2003). Instead, in this last section, I will suggest approaches, methods, and particular content that I feel are essential, or at least facilitative, to the transformative process which is the aim of an introductory course.

First and foremost, learning has to be viewed as a holistic process, involving the whole person, not just an intellectual enterprise. It is important to help students realize that there are multiple sources of knowledge, and to this end, multiple types of learning experiences need to be provided beyond the course readings and videos.

Students must combine their journey into the world of "others" with an in-depth reflection on their own cultural experience, particularly in their formative years and the "critical incidents" (Montalvo, 1999) that have had particular impact on their development and who they have become.

In the process, they will become aware of their "cultural lens," perhaps for the first time, and examine how this affects their own lives and their perceptions and interactions with others at the personal and professional levels. To this end, the most effective tool devised by my colleagues (Mitchell Maki, PhD, Joseph Nunn, PhD, and Jorja Leap, PhD) and I was the cultural autobiography assignment, an exploration of the impact of the student's cultural milieu across time guided by specific questions that helped provide insight into both the overt and more subtle and covert influences of their cultural experience. The writing of the cultural autobiography generally provided a cathartic, often dramatic, experience for the students and a breakthrough in perception, not only in reference to self, but to the impact of culture in anyone's life. Equally important, however, was the responses of the students' peers and the professor. Presenting a summary of the "findings" of this personal journey and its impact upon them to their peers created new bonds within the group based on a new appreciation of others' experiences that revealed a person often quite different and much more complex than expected and a sharing of similar experiences across individuals, even if the cultural context varied. For my part, I carried on a dialog with the student on paper, responding at length and in depth to the elements of self shared on the page. In many areas, I would ask questions or propose possibilities to explore further, in an attempt to nudge students to another level of insight. This was always done cautiously and sensitively, with the students understanding that their responses were for their benefit, not my curiosity, and that they could keep their written responses to themselves with the simple notation that they had answered them privately.

Students cannot learn about diversity without experiencing it directly with individuals culturally different from self. I have already discussed the first, relative safe step, beginning with one's peers. But for significant learning to occur, the students must move out of their university cohort and interact with "others" in the larger community. This needs to be on two levels, a community experience and an interpersonal dialog. The first requires the student to attend some community event sponsored by a cultural group other than his/her own. It is important that the student have the experience of being the "other" and learn to relate to persons and activities in a different milieu. It is essential that the students be required to obtain information from the participants, so that they are not passive by-standers and so that they understand their observations in the correct context. It is a given to make sure that students choose events that will offer them a positive experience.

The ethnographic interview is one of the most valuable learning experience in the course, particularly when it is used as shared material in the class or small group. The aim of the ethnographic interview is to obtain the "insider's" or emic view of the culture, as they see it reflected in the perspectives, views, beliefs, behavior, etc., of themselves and others in the culture they share. Spradley and McCurdy (1972) provide a thorough description and exemplary case examples from the perspective of sociologists; Green (1999) offers an excellent guide to the ethnographic interview and approach for the social work professional. It has been my experience that it is necessary to provide an interview schedule guide for the student, of broad open-ended questions that cover significant areas of the informant's cultural experience and interaction with mainstream society. This allows the students to compare and contrast experiences of various cultural groups given that parallel information is obtained. Finally, it is not only important to have the students share their ethnographic interview material with the class or group, but to reflect on and share with the group how the experience affected them, including the emotional impact and the correction of misconceptions. This sharing of ethnographies introduces the students to the insider's world of many different cultural groups.

First person narrative is a powerful learning tool. Because there is time for only one or two ethnographic interviews, the use of first person narratives is an excellent supplement that offers additional privy to worlds and perspectives different from one's own. For example, *Hearts of Sorrow* (Freeman, 1989) presents the accounts of Vietnamese refugees detailing their lives in Vietnam under Communist rule, the dangers of their escape with their families by boat, and their difficulties and successes in their adjustment in the U.S., all in their own words. To enhance the impact of the two stories I assign, I have the students write a narrative of their own as though they were a member of the family. (For additional details, see de Anda, in press.) Videos are particularly effective if they are first person narratives rather than documentaries presenting information from an outsider's (the camera's or narrator's) position. Congressman Ron Dellums describing before Congress his experience as a young child watching his Japanese American friend being loaded onto a truck and taken away to a relocation camp, the young Vietnamese adolescent describing his marginal existence as *bui doi* (dust of life), and the shared journey of a Jewish bi-sexual filmmaker and her born-again Christian brother as they struggle to try and understand each others' worlds, all create a uniquely empathic experience for the students.

Students need to understand that behavior occurs in a context and that observation alone, no matter how careful, does not always provide the information for accurate understanding. Students need to begin to move from behavior to understanding differences in perceptions of behavior, to the underlying assumptions upon which these perceptions are based, to the values that direct behavior and impact perceptions and assumptions. The same behaviors can mean very different things for different cultural groups and very different behaviors can indicate the same thing. For example, to make my point, I have asked my students how they greet an elder relative. They have given a range of responses from enthusiastic hugs and kisses to purposefully maintaining distance and bowing slightly, both as signs of respect and affection.

One must take care not to over-simplify and homogenize ethnic/cultural groups. The potential for this may be greater in introductory courses, where so much material has to be covered in order to present an adequate overview of diverse populations. Devore and Schlesinger (1981-1999) have emphasized this point for decades, indicating the importance of attending to the intersect of ethnicity and social class. Falicov (1995) has developed a model for viewing the individual as multidimensional even while recognizing the cultural context. This complexity is difficult to convey to the newcomer and must be re-emphasized and elaborated upon in subsequent courses.

It is important to employ both micro and macro perspectives and indicate the linkages between the two. To understand the issues of individuals and families employing the intersect of ethnicity/culture and social class requires an examination of societal, structural factors to move beyond a blame the victim (or the culture) stance. Moreover, it is important not to get trapped in "the blame game" (sometimes cloaked in the hunt for "responsibility"), which results from asking the wrong questions. Better questions to teach students to ask are: What contributed to the creation of this situation/condition? What contributes to its continuance and helps maintain it? What are the barriers to change? The concept of empowerment and an understanding of collaboration should be introduced as a natural progression in their search for the answers to these questions and their understanding of the impact of structural factors on the individual and groups.

An important example of the intersect of the micro and macro is the impact of historical events, particularly trauma, across generations. Historical events are not just something that occurs at one point in time; they can transform the individuals involved in profound ways that affect future generations in a multitude of ways, including intergenerational interactions, opportunities, perspectives, health and well-being, to name a few. The trauma of living through genocide is evident in the offspring of such diverse groups as American Indian, Jewish Holocaust, and Armenian genocide survivors. The legacy of the losses created by the American Indian boarding schools and the discrimination of Jim Crow laws affect subsequent generations.

The concept of privilege, particularly White privilege (MacIntosh, 1989), its various manifestations, and its direct contribution to the maintenance of discrimination and oppression need to be an integral part of the course. However, there are a number of pitfalls that must be avoided. First, it should not become the focus of the course, even in courses that have predominantly White students. Discerning and acknowledging the role of White privilege in their lives, while essential, should not become the centerpiece of the students' learning. The aim of the course is to recognize one's own cultural lens, but then move beyond to recognize the many other cultural lenses that exist and the commonalities and differences. Over-focusing on White privilege or making it an underlying framework for the course, in a sense, establishes privilege again, with examination of the privileged experience of the mainstream taking a larger role in a course that is supposed to be *multi*cultural. The intent can also backfire, at least initially, breeding guilt and defensiveness or self-protection that make students less likely to risk and share with their peers, thus interfering with the group learning process.

It is important to remember that the transformative process is not necessarily linear (Bourjolly et al., 2005) or that the pace may vary at times from epiphany to hesitation. Opportunities also need to be provided for integrating the learning materials, their group experience, and their community experiences, either as an assignment or a focused group process.

Finally, thought has to be given as to how to evaluate progress in the course that is consistent with the transformative aim of the course. Do standard grading procedures, both with regard to assignments and final grades, contribute to the learning process and accurately capture the student's progress? With regard to assignments, particularly the cultural autobiography, the ethnographic reports, and the first person narrative accounts, individualized feedback from the teacher is critical for validating what for most will be a unique learning experience. In my courses, this has often included giving the students a "grade" of R for revise and using their written word to create a Socratic dialog of sorts that will guide their revision. The paper that is finally evaluated is the result of this individualized interactive and reflective process. Finally, the readings in the course are not intended for memorization of detail to regurgitate in a quantifiable way. However, creative methods are needed to encourage students to complete the reading that will allow them to get the most from their classroom and community experiences and to contribute in their discussion groups.

CONCLUSION

The preceding observations and suggestions were made in relation to courses that serve as the students' first introduction to ethnic/cultural diversity. There are two caveats regarding the role of such courses in the curriculum. First, it is ill-conceived to have only one course that focuses specifically on diversity (diverse populations and related issues), no matter how well designed or apparently comprehensive. This is the case for a number of reasons: (1) It gives the erroneous message that everything significant about diverse populations and cultures can be neatly packaged and learned in a short period of time (a sort of "Everything you ever wanted to know about–fill in the group–but were too P.C. to ask"), (2) It doesn't convey the extent to which this knowledge is critical for all aspects of the profession: direct practice, policy, and research, (3) It results in either overwhelming the students with material or running the risk of presenting general overviews that may contribute rather than work to debunk stereotypes, (4) It limits the amount of time needed for individual and group processing which is basic to learning and personal and professional growth in this area. This is not to imply that a single course cannot have a significant impact on student knowledge and growth, but that limiting it to one course also limits the potential for students' development.

Second, the learning achieved in this introductory course needs to be reinforced by the *prominence* of diversity content in other courses in the curriculum if the message of its important is to ring true. This means that diversity content is clearly integrated in other courses, not just a few obligatory articles appended to the syllabus or, worse, the same case materials used with different ethnic names attached and issues presented and discussed acontextually.

The emphasis in this article has been on ethnic and cultural diversity, given the focus of the journal; however, the MSW courses I have taught have always included populations in the broader CSWE mandate, particularly with regard to sexual orientation, disability, and religion. Most of the observations apply to these populations as well, and consideration of these groups also intersects with ethnicity and social class in a multidimensional approach.

The aim of this article was to present some observations that might be useful for those designing introductory courses on diversity. The task is particularly challenging, fraught with the potential disinterest of students fulfilling a curriculum requirement or hostility and resistance from students threatened by the unfamiliar. However, given the proper learning environment in the classroom and revelatory experiences in the community beyond, it can also be a uniquely rewarding learning experience for both the students and the teacher.

REFERENCES

Bourjolly, J. N., Sands, R. G., Solomon, P., Stanhope, V., Pernell-Arnold, A., and Finley, L. (2005). The journey towards intercultural sensitivity: A non-linear process. *Journal of Ethnic & Cultural Diversity in Social Work,* 14(3/4), 41-62.

de Anda, D. (1984). Bicultural socialization: Factors affecting the minority experience. *Social Work,* March-April, 101-107.

de Anda, D. (in press). Teaching social work with multicultural populations: A holistic approach to learning. *Journal of Teaching in Social Work.*

Devore, W., and Schlesinger, E. (1981, 1987, 1991, 1995, 1999). *Ethnic sensitive social work practice,* Boston, MA: Allyn & Bacon.

Falicov, C. (1995). Training to think culturally: A multidimensional comparative framework. *Family Process,* 34, 373-389.

Freeman, J. M. (1989). *Hearts of sorrow.* Stanford, CA: Stanford University Press.

Garcia, B., and Van Soest, D. (2000). Facilitating learning on diversity: Challenges to the professor. *Journal of Ethnic & Cultural Diversity in Social Work,* 9(1/2), 21-39.

Green, J. W. (1982, 1995, 1999). *Cultural awareness in the human services.* Needham Heights, MA: Allyn & Bacon.

Lee, M. Y., and Greene, G. J. (2003). A teaching framework for transformative multicultural social work education. *Journal of Ethnic & Cultural Diversity in Social Work,* 12(3), 1-28.

Lum, D. (Ed.). (1999, 2003). *Culturally competent practice.* Pacific Grove, CA: Brooks/Cole–Thomson Learning.

McIntosh, P. (1989). White privilege: Unpacking the invisible knapsack. *Peace and Freedom,* July/August, 10-12.

Mezirow, J., and Associates. (Eds.). (2000). *Learning as transformation: Critical perspectives on a theory in progress.* San Francisco, CA: Jossey-Bass.

Montalvo, F. F. (1999). The critical incident interview and ethnoracial identity. *Journal of Multicultural Social Work,* 7(3/4), 19-43.

Spradley, J. P., and Mc Curdy, D. W. (1972). *The cultural experience: Ethnography in complex society.* Chicago, IL: Science Research Associates, Inc.

Creating a Diverse Spiritual Community: Reflections from a Spirituality and Social Work Practice Class

Sherri F. Seyfried

INTRODUCTION

This summer, I had one of the most rewarding teaching experiences when I taught a six week elective graduate course entitled, *Spirituality and Social Work Practice*. I had a similar experience when I first taught the class two years ago. However, this experience was more profound; perhaps the second time around I gained more "wisdom," and I was more comfortable with the subject matter. I am sure these were contributing factors, but there was something qualitatively different about the "collective experience." This class was more diverse than the first class, diverse in terms of race, ethnicity, religion, age, life experiences, spiritual beliefs, and values. It was the diversity in student experience that created the range in the exchange of ideas while at the same time creating the space for us to experience and mirror common human qualities. Through our diverse world views evolved interdependence and spiritual kinship.

Giving myself some time to step back and reflect upon the class experience, I am able to identify the processes and group dynamics that enabled this diverse spiritual community to unfold. As we prepare students to advocate against discrimination and to promote social justice, how well prepared are they to meet these challenges they will face in today's socio-political economy? They will need to draw on personal and interpersonal resources to refuel the compassion needed for the challenges ahead, compassion rooted in meaning and purpose that moves beyond self. Towards this effort, what responsibility as social work educators do we have in creating the space for students to find and sustain greater meaning and connection to the profession's traditional core values? This essay represents my reflections on how a diverse spiritual community was formed and concludes with implications for social work education.

BACKGROUND

There were 24 part time students in the class, with the overwhelming majority of them working full time jobs. Half of the students had just completed their first year in the foundation with the other half just completing the second year of the foundation. This course is designed to explore the concept of "spirituality" as it relates to the profession of social work and provides a holistic perspective to guide professional social work practice. The course emphasizes the distinction between religion and spirituality, which was a recurrent theme throughout the course.

Canda and Furman (1999) refer to religion as an ". . . institutionalized pattern of beliefs, behavior, and experiences, oriented toward spiritual concerns and shared by a community and transmitted over time in tradition" (p. 42). The authors go on to explain spirituality as a sense of meaning, purpose, and connectedness that is not necessarily associated with any particular institution. Spirituality has more to do with what it means to be human, a synthesis of the biological, psychological, spiritual, and physical dimensions that together make us whole. Religion is externally located whereas spirituality is internally located.

Each evening after class, when the students and I walked to our cars, we would comment on our overwhelming sense of calm and tranquility. But more importantly, we felt what we were experiencing was connected to something bigger than any one of us. Students noticed that in work and in class they were more focused, creative, and they were not as distracted by everyday hassles. It has been documented elsewhere that contemplative practices enhance the learning process and are complementary to critical thinking (Hart, 2004). Students also commented that family members noticed something was "different" about them. Students commented that they learned so much from each other. Student evaluations and reflection papers echoed similar sentiments. We had created a space where we could, as one student stated, ". . . relate to the humaneness in each other;" ". . . we don't often have the opportunity for that kind of experience."

ESTABLISHING "RELATIONAL SPIRITUALITY"

It was important to create an environment where students would feel comfortable taking risks. Creating a safe environment that encourages value clarification is fundamental to spiritual growth (Canda & Furman, 1999). Towards that effort, we set a few preliminary ground rules: (1) We would not "debate," but we would "dialogue." (2) We determined what happens in the class stays in the class. (3) We would respect diverse opinions and experiences. Rather than sit in the traditional classroom structure with one row behind the other, we sat in a circle so we could face each other. This seating arrangement helped to personalize the dialogue. I abandoned the use of Power Point; using it would have taken focus away from the group. To some extent this was a metaphor for letting go of the "power" that professors typically hold in the "traditional" classroom.

Contemplative exercises like meditation, guided imagery, and poetry were used to facilitate intrapersonal and interpersonal awareness. On most evenings, we began the class with some form of meditation to help us center and focus so we could be more aware of "the here and now" and living in the moment (Hahn, 1975). Early on in the class, we had a poetry night where we shared our favorite poem and spoke about the poem's importance for us. What I thought would be an evening of mutual reflection turned out to be an evening of cathartic expression, connection, and feeling. Something had happened to connect us in a very profound way. The poems were a reflection of what was important to us, how we saw the world, our hopes, and our dreams. Some students chose to read religious scriptures from the bible; others chose poems that represented their cultural frame of reference; some chose poems that talked of friendship, and other students chose poems reflecting spiritual meaning and purpose. It was at the conclusion of this evening that the class formed a sense of interdependence or "relational spirituality" (Faver, 2004). In reference to relational spirituality, Krieglstein (2006) states,

> entering into relationships, into the reality of others, involves recognizing our need for other people whose perspectives complement, challenge, and expand our own. Relational spirituality has relevance for individual growth, forming relationships with our clients, and is consonant with social work values and ethics, i.e., respecting the client's right to self determination, and respect for diversity (p. 27).

The poetry night enabled us to relate to each other in a very basic human way. We felt a sense of trust and acceptance, that it was okay to be vulnerable and share a glimpse into that "inner core" that makes us who we are. It was at this point that the dance between intrapersonal and interpersonal spiritual development began to evolve. We were ready for the "real learning" to take place; we had formed the beginnings of a spiritual community. Diana Chapman Walsh (2006) makes reference to a speech Elie Wiesel delivered at Wellesley College wherein he presents a vision of a community that enables honoring of diverse values: ". . . he described a moral society–or a community striving to be moral–as one that is living in dialogue, that is honoring the humanity of every member. In such a community we are all lifelong learners, teachers, and witnesses" (p. 123). Regardless of the context in which we find ourselves, either at work, home, or in the community, when we are in spiritual relationship, we allow ourselves to become learners, teachers or witnesses. Each role provides a portal for us to learn something about ourselves in relation to the "other"; this is what it means to fully embrace diversity. While it is important to *value* diversity, obtain *knowledge* about diverse populations, or increase diversity by the "*numbers,*" these efforts alone do not move us towards interdependence. Interdependence is about "being" in relation with the "other."

EXAMPLES OF INTERDEPENDENCE

As the class began to relate to each other in a mindful way, there were a number of instances that illustrated interdependence and connectedness. I will share a few of them here. When we were making plans for a Native American guest speaker to visit the class, a Native American student shared with the class that in her culture it is customary to give a gift when someone does something for you. She suggested that we all bring a small gift and the following week she would bring a basket in which we could place the gifts. We were all in agreement and brought the gifts the following week. What happened after that was most interesting. I noticed every week from that time forward, one or two students would bring some type of food to share with the entire class. This was not organized. I don't believe there was even any conversation about bringing food. We consciously or unconsciously decided it was important to share with one another. This experience provides a material example of interdependence. However, there were also numerous exchanges that represented examples of non-material interdependence. Students were very respectful of other students who were openly questioning their belief system. For extrinsically oriented students, this questioning usually began with unconscious expressions of anger and frustration. Class members responded with objective compassion that allowed the space for continued re-evaluation and introspection.

GUEST LECTURERS AND THEIR ROLE IN BUILDING RELATIONAL SPIRITUALITY

Invited guest lecturers were also central to the development of relational spirituality. Each guest spoke from "the heart." One guest, a visual artist and writer, spoke about "spirituality in the arts." She shared with the class a poem that was inspired from a dream she had at a time of transition in her life. The poem was about her journey in pursuing a dream and the uncertainty of not knowing what lay ahead. She later had a videographer create a visual image of her poem. Her presentation evoked a range of responses. One student stated, "I never really thought about art in this way." For other students, she helped to rekindle creative expression that was dormant. "I used to love to paint, until one day someone said your work is awful; you should never paint again." A personal transformation began to occur for this student, not only in a renewed interest in painting, but a new perspective about "self."

Another guest speaker shared her experiences growing up on a reservation in the Northeast. She spoke of the discrimination she experienced growing up as well as her later experiences as an urban Native American. Students of Haitian descent identified with the speaker's experience of bi-culturalization: "I too celebrate cultural practices that are a part of my Haitian heritage while at the same time also incorporating traditional religious practices (Catholicism) that are a result of European domination." Another guest speaker, an Episcopalian priest and social worker, spoke about spirituality and homosexuality. Extrinsically oriented students were very challenged by his presentation; for them "spirituality" and "homosexuality" had contradictory meanings. He met their cynicism and skepticism with such compassion and love. For other students, his presentation was very affirming. His patience and compassion created a space conducive to dialogue and introspection.

Each guest lecturer brought a unique perspective to spirituality which contributed to the depth and breadth of our spiritual awareness. But more importantly, it was the guests' level of compassion towards their work and sense of interdependence that contributed to the experience as a whole and to individual student growth.

The context of the spirituality class provided the "ideal" context in which to build a diverse spiritual community. Many of the steps taken were deliberate, while others were unanticipated. In the beginning of the class, it was apparent that the traditional classroom setup and pedagogy would not facilitate an environment conducive to spiritual growth, creativity, and interdependence; therefore, it was necessary to "let go" of some of the authority. If faculty, social workers, and administrators are to have the vision to establish communities based upon spiritual principles and values, then it will be necessary for those in authority to re-evaluate their roles in relation to creating that vision. Equally important is to gain a "way of knowing" that connects work, habitude, and spirituality.

IMPLICATIONS FOR SOCIAL WORK EDUCATION

There is a growing interdisciplinary movement for the integration of contemplative practices in higher education and in the workplace (Awbrey et al., 2006; Faver, 2004; Kriger, 2006; Lindholm & Astin,

2006; Zajonc, 2006). This movement is largely led by academics who believe we need another way of "knowing" that leads to transformative, holistic learning. They are concerned about the world in which we live. In our society, there is a prevailing sense of disconnectedness. There is a schism in humanity that is continuing to polarize groups of individuals, "them vs US." We see this phenomenon being played out in the media and in the workplace; yet we feel hopeless to do anything about it. Capra (1997) states there are solutions to these complex problems; however, they require a radical shift in how we see the world and in our values. He states that most individuals with leadership positions in higher education and in the workplace have not come to the realization that this shift is *needed* for our *survival.*

Historically the Social Work profession has had a core set of values and ethics based upon Judeo-Christian beliefs. However, I don't believe we have fully developed our *thinking* about what it means to apply them in relation to the political, economic, and cultural realities of our society. These core values are: (1) service, (2) social justice, (3) dignity and worth of the person, (4) importance of human relationships, (5) integrity, and (6) competence. More recently, CSWE has issued a mandate that spirituality must be a part of the curriculum. How this content is incorporated into the curriculum and applied to social work practice varies by each School of Social Work. More thought is needed regarding the associations between the profession's core values, spirituality, and social advocacy.

ENVISIONING A REALISTIC AND COMPASSIONATE PRACTICE FOR SOCIAL JUSTICE

Houston (2002) claims that while the Social Work profession values social justice, we have few models that help us with the realities associated with *practicing social justice.* Students will work as clinicians and as administrators. Many will work in large public, bureaucratic organizations facing major budget cuts, fewer resources, with more demands for accountability. Disproportionate numbers of poor individuals and families of color are being served in these large public agencies. Houston (2002) provides a model of cultural practice that simultaneously acknowledges the structural inequalities that maintain oppression *and* the political and cultural factors within bureaucratic organizations that influence the social worker's (and client's) sense of agency. While Houston's model helps us with the *doing* or *how to* part of social advocacy, it will take a certain resolve, compassion, creativity, and maturity to carry through with this type of practice.

In the spirituality class, we discussed the formal and informal policies, organizational culture, and politics that impede advocacy efforts. Classmates offered creative solutions they have used to navigate the "system." What I noticed is that the students who volunteered personal examples of their advocacy efforts were also the students who appeared to have strong spiritual identities. They were very compassionate about advocacy; they were older, and had more years of work experience. In other words, these students were *doing* and *being* what it means to advocate for social justice. They were confident in their actions; they found *meaning* and *purpose* in their work that extended beyond self. For them work and spirituality were inseparable; spirituality wasn't something practiced at home; it was a part of their total being. Not all students, regardless of age, have reached this level of spiritual growth.

As we prepare students to become professional social workers, if we are to remain true to the profession's traditional values in today's trying times, we (students and educators) will need to attend to intrapersonal and interpersonal spiritual development that enables us to relate humanely to others, spiritual development that extends beyond our own self interests. In our spirituality class, we experienced being part of a diverse spiritual community; it was important for us to be able to know and feel what the possibilities could be. However, this learning is sustained when students see the possibilities of relational spirituality modeled in other places in the program. Students are very observant of the organizational dynamics within institutions; they see what is valued and not valued. These observations can be powerful influences. Diana Chapman Walsh (2006) quoting Gandhi, states "we need to *be* the change we want to see" if we are to help students find meaning and purpose that extends beyond self. She goes on to say that faculty and others in leadership positions should be "self-conscious about the values we enact day to day."

In our classrooms, amongst our colleagues in the academy, and in the workplace, we need to be *mindful* that our actions and dialogue create space for inquiry, creativity, diverse perspectives, and growth. This type of community fosters interdependence, connectedness, meaning, and purpose that extend beyond self interests. This type of community creates the "synergy" needed to develop creative visions of what can be.

REFERENCES

Awbrey, S., Dana, D., Miller, V., Robinson, P., Ryan, M., & Scott, D. (Eds.). (2006). *Integrative learning and action: A call to wholeness.* New York: Peter Lang.

Canda, Edward R., & Furman, L. (1999). *Spiritual diversity in social work practice: The heart of helping.* New York: Free Press.

Capra, F. (1997). *The web of life: A new understanding of living systems.* New York: Double-day.

Faver, C. (2004). Relational spirituality and social caregiving. *Social Work, 49*(2), 241-249.

Hahn, T. N. (1987). *The miracle of mindfulness: An introduction to the practice of meditation.* Boston: Beacon Press.

Hart, T. (2004). Opening the contemplative mind in the classroom. *Journal of Transformative Education, 2*(1), 28-46.

Houston, S. (2002). Reflecting on habitus, field and capital: Towards a culturally sensitive social work. *Journal of Social Work. 2,* 146-167.

Kreieglstein, M. (2006). Spirituality and Social Work. *Dialogue and Universalism, 5* 1-10.

Kriger, M. (2006). Ways of questioning that can transform organizations and people. In D. S. Awbrey, V. Miller, P. Robinson, M. Ryan, & D. Scott (Eds.), *Integrative learning and action: A call to wholeness* (pp. 199-217). New York: Peter Lang.

Lindholm, J. A., & Astin, H. S. (2006). Understanding the "Interior" life of faculty: How important is spirituality? *Religion and Education, 33*(2), 64-90.

Walsh, D. C. (2006). The search for meaning and uncommon values. In D. S. Awbrey, V. Miller, P. Robinson, M. Ryan, & D. Scott (Eds.), *Integrative learning and action: A call to wholeness* (pp. 117-128). New York: Peter Lang.

Zajonc, A. (2006). Science and spirituality: Finding the right map. In D. S. Awbrey, V. Miller, P. Robinson, M. Ryan, & D. Scott (Eds.), *Integrative learning and action: A call to wholeness* (pp. 57-80). New York: Peter Lang.

REFLECTIONS ON THE IMPACT OF STRUCTURAL FORCES ON OUR CLIENTS AND OURSELVES

Disparity/Inequity, Knowledge Production and Public Policy

Ruth Enid Zambrana
John K. Holton

INTRODUCTION

The two authors combined have 50 years of experience in developing knowledge (research), applying knowledge (practice), and observing how policy is implemented through public systems. Our observations and experience inform this essay on racial and ethnic health disparities and child health and well-being. Our intent in this essay is twofold: to argue that the tools of social science and public health research rarely are used to challenge the contemporary arrangements of our social structure and, secondly, to underscore approaches for research that remain under-examined and unexplored.

From time to time, social science research finds its way back into relevancy. Its analytical tools are capable of critiquing current social policy that masks institutional racism, as in racial profiling (Knowles, Persico, & Todd, 2001), or explaining why crime does not occur in neighborhoods populated with the usual demographic suspects of income, unemployment, and minorities (Sampson, Raudenbush, & Earls, 1997), or whether home visiting services can deter child maltreatment and fatal injuries (Donovan et al., 2007). Lately, social science is encouraging adoption of "evidence-based" certification based almost exclusively on randomized trials as the *nom de guerre* for social work related practices (Chaffin & Friedrich, 2004; Mullen & Streiner, 2004). In its loftier moments toward influencing social applications of knowledge, public health and social science research anoint services as "promising/proven practices" or tag initiatives with "best practice" labels.

A closer look at the fields of social science and public health and their scientific discourse reveals something less celebratory and more disturbing, namely the absence of clarity and the proliferation of old understandings as "new" discoveries. Take for instance the subject of disparity. *Disparity* is now the new jargon in science to define or imply a measurable and statistical difference between two events (USDHHS, 2005). Disparity replaces inequity as the term of choice in our literature. Hence, the U.S. Department of Health and Human Services (2006) does not use the term inequity because it may (1) imply an ethical judgment about differences; (2) is not unambiguously measurable or observable; and most importantly, (3) involves judgments about what a society believes is *unfair*. So what is fair?

Reflecting on health disparities and the differences found among African American, Latino, and Non-Hispanic White groups, we are left with the inevitable task of deciphering the very meaning of this "new" terminology. What are the underlying assumptions that will guide the drive to reduce or eliminate health disparities? What are we as a society willing to do when we uncover or rediscover the factors that are associated with disparities?

IMPLICIT ASSUMPTIONS IN THE RESEARCH ENTERPRISE

Research is guided by implicit moral roadmaps, which are defined as neutral or objective theoretical frameworks and methodologies, but which provide information that is explicitly subjective and shapes our views of population groups and fairness. The culture of science which claims to embody blind neutrality, empiricism, and positivist thinking has embarked on a long journey to reproduce old knowledge as new knowledge. The meaning and interpretation of the numerous studies on poverty and all the other veiled names that include low-income, poor, culture, disparity, inequality, and social gradient have to be challenged with respect to science or knowledge production and its link to public policy. These are some roadmaps which in our view continue the reproduction of knowledge that works against policy changes:

- Implicit assumptions of individual agency and an equal playing field prevent researchers from identifying the intersections of institutional racism, poverty, gender and the associations of these factors with the domains of individual well-being, health outcomes, and racial/ethnic disparities.
- Cultural determinism is a panacea in science to ascribe both positive and negative attributes that makes outcomes non-modifiable and unchangeable. For example, the Hispanic health epidemiologic paradox argues that Latinos have better outcomes despite low SES because their culture endorses strong social support and nutritious dietary patterns. When the outcomes are bad, it is also due to Latino culture that encourages avoidance of health care services and sedentary practices. These discourses are both uninformed and continue to maintain systems of inequality in place.
- The culture of science proffers all issues related to race, ethnicity, and SES as a conundrum–it is complex or mysterious when the

conditions of darker "races" are examined and somehow approachable and solvable for other non-racialized groups.
*   The uncontested politics of knowledge production are visible, that is, who is funded and who is included as research principals and research subjects. For example, the NIH Institute for Research on Women has allocated more than $600 million over the last 15 years for women's health in major disease conditions such as cardiovascular disease and osteoporosis. Few, if any, African American and Latino women participated as principals, and data on those at the highest risk of premature disability and mortality, namely African American and Latino women with respect to CVD, breast cancer, hypertension, and diabetes, are under-explored.

Poverty and its consequences have been discussed in encyclopedic magnitude in the scientific literature. We know, or at least we write as if we know, that impoverished environments harm children, cripple families, and stagnate communities. We know that poor children find themselves slipping on wobbly flooring and see a rapidly descending ceiling on their dreams. We have interviewed enough parents and primary caregivers to know that it is their desperate hopes which allow us entry into their homes for longitudinal and cross-sectional data gathering (in contrast to the resistance and reluctance from middle-class and higher cohorts). We know also that the best analyses of poverty almost always include a penetrating assessment of the confounding presence of race/ethnicity. Yet when the smoke clears, we seldom read a critique of status quo components that structure salaries, residence, education, and access to the pipelines for a better life. The knowledge is abundant, the will to challenge policy assumptions and budgets tepid. What is worrisome is that policy decisions continue to mandate research while children continue to suffer under public systems of safety, housing, education and health that intersect to affect access to–and quality of–child health outcomes.

CHILD HEALTH, POVERTY, AND PUBLIC POLICY

Lets take an example. *Children's Health, The Nation's Wealth: Assessing Children's Health* (2004), an Institute of Medicine (IOM) report, provides a detailed examination of the information about children's health that is needed to help policy makers and program providers at the federal, state, and local levels. In order to improve children's health–and, thus, the health of future generations–it is critical to have data that can be used to assess both current conditions and possible future threats to children's health. This compelling report describes what is known about the health of children and what is needed to expand the knowledge. By strategically improving the health of children, we ensure healthier future generations to come. Children's health has clearly improved over the past several decades. Significant and positive gains have been made in lowering rates of infant mortality and morbidity from infectious diseases and accidental causes, improved access to health care, and reduction in the effects of environmental contaminants such as lead. Yet the report asserts that major questions still remain about how to assess the status of children's health, what factors should be monitored, and the appropriate measurement tools that should be used. (Institute of Medicine, www.iom.edu/cms, accessed May 29, 2007)

The IOM report calls for additional research, a new definition of child health, and coordination and integration of federal, state, and local data systems to link individual data across data sets. It is a laudable report, albeit several issues were raised without answers. It states that worrisome outcomes by race, ethnic, and SES groups remain a *mystery*. It also shows again a worsening of our place internationally on several indicators. The report raises questions about how data should be used to inform policy and practice. If reports are scientifically based, are they not intended to yield new ways to solve issues and policy to support new solutions? If "change" is needed, how do we incorporate information of the last 100 years? What are the purposes of these reports? Who monitors? What do they monitor? As welcomed as the IOM report was for its courage and forthrightness of presentation, we raise these concerns as the catalyst for new directions in social science and public health research. A prominent question is–do we know enough about factors associated with child well-being and child health to change or institutionalize policies and services? Or, stated differently, what do we know that can help direct knowledge acquisition?

1. First and foremost, we know that poverty matters, because it is associated with economic instability and stress, poor nutrition, limited access to quality resources (education, health, recreational, and mental health). Secondly, we cannot look at children without placing them within context of families. Resources available within communities are the key variables for scientific examination.
2. Race and ethnicity matter. Race/ethnicity cannot be used alone to analyze data as its meaning is best understood in the interrelationship of race/ethnicity and poverty. These meanings are mediated

by the seemingly invisible dual service systems in education, health, criminal justice, mortgage lending, and insurance to name only a few.

3. Community matters. The after-school activities, the safety of the community, the police, the recreational facilities, and the responsiveness of the public and private institutions in those communities where children live greatly influence their well-being. Hyper-racial and economic segregation is associated with limited allocation of resources and poor quality of services.

4. Inequity in access to social and economic resources in those communities that are most disadvantaged prevent the development of economically viable and healthy communities.

Returning to the topic of poverty, we cannot hope to solve the problem without examining and quantifying variables that represent structural arrangements that produce disparities and inequities. We would argue that research questions such as, "What role does a child born into poverty play in the maintenance of his/her economic and educational disparity?" are less compelling to pursue than these: "How does our market economy maintain the status quo of economic, health, employment, and educational inequality and disparity?" "Is the informal (i.e., "good old boys") network capable of being revamped and updated given the challenges of post modern diversity represented by new elites (women and individuals of color)?"

PUBLIC SYSTEMS AS SITES OF INEQUITY AND PRODUCTION OF INEQUALITY

In today's neo-liberal governance, public systems serve as gate-keepers rather than safety nets of resources to help groups or vulnerable populations who need it most. Persistent discriminatory patterns within public systems favor Non-Hispanic White groups over African American, Latino, and Native American populations. In recent reviews of empirical and historical work on major public systems, namely welfare, education and civic participation, persistent historical and contemporary patterns of exclusionary and inequitable forms of implementation of policy were found (Dill et al., 2004; Noguera, 2003; Silliman, Fried, Ross, & Gutierrez, 2004). This calls into question the execution of the original intent of the 1964 Civil Rights legislation that was passed initially as a remedy for the unequal treatment of historically under-represented groups and women to "level the playing field." Two decades later this legislation transformed from a specific intent to a broader, all-inclusive intent of diversity that essentially masks the persistent and unequal distribution of resources to low-income African American and Latino groups. This new intent may be similar to what Zuberi (2001) calls statistical racism, whereby race is used as an independent variable or contributor to an outcome without taking into account the role of social processes. He observes "A true human science will necessarily investigate population experiences within the broader context of society" (p. xxi).

For the past several decades, health care research has begun to focus on complex, historical, multifaceted racial and ethnic disparities, as documented by another Institute of Medicine (IOM) report, *Unequal Treatment: Confronting Racial and Ethnic Disparities in Health Care* (2003). The report reviewed over 800 studies that showed a link between poverty, unequal treatment, and adverse outcomes (chronic conditions, earlier mortality, greater morbidity) and concluded that racial and ethnic minorities receive inferior quality of care compared with their non-Hispanic White counterparts, even after controlling for insurance status and socioeconomic status. Are these ideas new? What is the *mystery* other than knowing that disciplines are not in conversation with one another and are reluctant to take on variables of self-exposure such as an examination of "provider culture, system culture, and science culture?"

When the first author recently attended a meeting at the National Academy of Sciences in Washington, DC, she noticed this quote by Albert Einstein (1879-1955) on the wall outside the building: "The Right to Search for Truth Implies also Duty: One Must Not Conceal Any Part Of What One Has Recognized To Be True." Yet the scholarship in social science, biomedical science, and public health science in so many ways conceals the truth. Some observations antithetical to Einstein's thinking about truth are these: Failure to acknowledge the intersections of equity or allocation of resources with quality available public service systems that can contribute to multiple life chances and opportunities for social engagement and upward mobility. Failure to acknowledge links which compound deficits among public service systems in housing, welfare, education, health, juvenile and criminal justice so that adverse outcomes for poor and historically underrepresented groups are viewed as individual or group failures rather than system failures.

After the release of this landmark 2003 IOM report, it would seem reasonable to assume that we would have moved beyond investing money into the production of old knowledge. Yet five years later the following headlines appeared in major public health publications:

- *Federal Report Examines Links Between Poverty, Health Access* (March 2007, p. 6)
- *High Rates of Incarcerated Black Men Devastating to Family Health* (March 2007, p. 6)
- *Knowing Family History Can Help Save Lives* (February 2007, p. 28)
- *Americans Rank Obesity as Top Health Issue for Children* (February 2007, p. 28)
- *US Preventive Care Lagging, Especially Among Minorities* (Source: Nation's Health, The official newspaper of the American Public Health Association, March 2007).

Similar headlines have also appeared in materials from many other professional associations, including the American Sociological Association.

We argue that racial and cultural attribution models that ignore key structural factors that construct racialized policies that disadvantage Latino and African American women and men must be continuously challenged. We argue that a disparity is not an individualized construct, but one formed by historical events and maintained by political governance.

The relationship between governance, social sciences, and production of knowledge is too cozy when dealing with issues of inequality and inequity, and the results seek to befuddle and dismiss underlying variables that capture historical, structural, and political forces that shape the experiences of those who experience disparity. For example, recent work on Mexican American women and higher education shows a clear historical model of staggered inequality. "Social utility" arguments emerged as appropriate rationales for permitting non-Hispanic White (NHW) women access to higher learning in the late eighteenth and early nineteenth centuries, and it was NHW women who first accessed private and public institutions in the 1970's and 1980's (Nash, 2005). Historicizing access to higher education demonstrates how hegemonic power has shaped access to educational institutions for African American and Mexican American women. These historical patterns are embedded and reproduced in the educational pipeline post Civil Rights legislation.

Significant reports and studies have been conducted over the last three decades by such well-known organizations as Chapin Hall in Chicago, National Center on Children and Poverty in New York, Foundation for Child Development, and, more recently, the Brookings Institute, Washington,

DC. In addition to this large generation of research, we are also informed about best practice approaches to child health from an interdisciplinary perspective–medicine, public health, sociology, and psychology which led to the implementation of programs such as Healthy Start/Healthy Families America, State Children's Health Insurance Program (SCHIP), and Head Start–all shown to be important to children's health.

Yet "new" reports constantly reset the national agenda, distract researchers and professionals from the known core issues of social inequality, and initiate redundant research initiatives that essentially reinvent the "I do not know" syndrome. We know that children need adequate housing, quality schools, good nutrition, and parents who have health insurance and living wage. If we provide this, we can then start a new generation of research that could yield some new data on child functioning and potential. We cannot expect different outcomes for children and historically under-represented groups when the material conditions of their lives remain the same.

CONCLUDING COMMENTS

When examining benchmark reports, existing public policy initiatives, and new research directions in areas such as child and adult obesity, chronic conditions or preventing child abuse, under-explored research questions are associated with the intersections of disparity and equity How can we generate new knowledge production if the conditions that contribute to the findings of disparity remain the same? Most importantly, why is not public policy being implemented based on the knowledge that conditions of poverty have antecedent variables such as illiteracy, unsafe neighborhoods, economic barriers to purchasing healthy food, and lack of health insurance, which exacerbate the impact of environmental hazards and poor quality health care? Although there are a plethora of public policy recommendations to address disparities in health, education, juvenile and criminal justice, child welfare, and employment, the standards of fairness serve to filter how much remedy is deserved.

Research in public health and social science is by definition reactive, that is, seldom does it identify social problems, more rarely does it accurately predict resolutions to our challenging issues. A better approach for social science research is to serve as our society's constitutional auditor. When science acts to "check the books" on equality and "justice for all," it goes beyond the convenience sampling of poor people to explain phenomena. For its sake, the scientific enterprise of learning, truth seeking, and knowledge production has to consider all the links in our society's chain or implode as a stagnating, self-serving edifice to maintain the status quo.

REFERENCES

Chaffin, M. and Friedrich, B. (2004). Evidence-based treatments in child abuse and neglect. *Children and Youth Services Review* 26, 1097-1113.

Donovan, E.F., Ammerman, R.T., Besl, J., Atherton, H., Khoury, J.C., Altaye, M., Putnam, F.W., and Van Ginkel, J.B. (2007). Intensive home visiting is associated with decreased risk of infant death. *Pediatrics* 119, 1124-1151.

Institute of Medicine (2003). Committee on Understanding and Eliminating racial and Ethnic Disaprities in Health Care. *Unequal treatment: Confroting racial and ethnic disparities in health care.* Washington, DC: The National Academies Press.

Jones-DeWeever, A., Dill, B.T., and Schram, S.F. (in press). Racial, ethnic and gender disparities in access to jobs, education and training under welfare reform. In B.T. Dill and R.E. Zambrana (Eds.), *Emerging Intersections: Race, Class, and Gender in Theory, Policy and Practice.* New Jersey: Rutgers University Press.

Knowles, J., Persico, N., and Todd, P. (2001). Racial bias in motor vehicle searches: Theory and evidence. *Journal of Political Economy* 109(1), 203-29.

Mullen, E.J. and Streiner, D.L. (2004). The evidence for and against evidence-based practice. *Brief Treatment and Crisis Intervention* 4(2), 111-121.

Nash, M. (2005). *Women's education in the United States, 1780-1840.* New York: Palgrave/Macmillan.

Noguera, P. (2003). *City Schools and the American Dream.* New York, NY: Teachers College Press.

Sampson, R., Raudenbush, S., and Earls, F. (1997). Neighborhoods and violent crime: A multilevel study of collective efficacy. *Science* 27, 918-924.

Silliman, J., Fried, M.G., Ross, L., and Gutierrez, E. (2004). *Undivided rights: Women of color organize for reproductive justice.* Cambrridge, MA: South End Press.

US Department of Health and Human Services (2005). *National Healthcare Disparities Report.* Agency for Healthcare Research and Quality. Rockville, MD.

US Department of Health and Human Services (2006). *National Healthcare Disparities Report.* Agency for Healthcare Research and Quality. Rockville, MD.

Zuberi, T. (2001). *Thicker than blood: How racial statistics lie.* Minneapolis, MN: University of Minnesota Press.

Reflections on Meanings and Applications of Social Justice

Rita Takahashi

SOCIAL JUSTICE MEANINGS

Word Usage

Social justice is the foundation of social work practice, and it is core to many community-based organizations, educational institutions, and professional associations and councils. Its value and significance to the social work profession are revealed in mission statements, codes of ethics, standards for accreditation, and principles and guidelines for social work practice.

Despite its prevalent use, social justice is seldom addressed in terms of definitions, specific goals, implementation, results, and evaluations. On one hand, it is frequently addressed as a desirable concept to which one should aspire; yet it is most often left nebulous and undefined. Many assume that others know what they mean by social justice, but if one inquires, one realizes that there are many vague perspectives and perceptions about what it is and how it is or should be manifested.

Social justice is identified by many educational institutions as a positive goal or mission. Although identified as something to be worked toward, seldom are the means for achievement or evidence for results identified. "What is social justice?" one wonders as one reads mission statements with these embedded words. "What are the forms of social justice?" "How does one know when social justice is achieved?" "What evidence points toward social justice?" These are but a few questions that arise as the term is commonly and freely used.

I have been a social work educator for almost 30 years, and during that time, I have seen expanding use of the term. I have been fascinated by the fact that few question what it means, even if the situation calls for it. For example, some schools of social work specify social justice in their mission; yet there is little explication as to how the goal for its achievement is instituted. Many simply assume that everyone knows what it means and that there is but one unified definition that remains static and stable through time. Actually, social justice is evolutionary, contextual, cultural, and fluid.

Definitions

The literature reveals many definitions of social justice that focus on means (processes) to ends (results). Folger and Cropanzano (1998) identify three types of justice, which they label interactional, procedural, and distributive. About the concept of justice, they say:

> Justice is about how rewards and punishments are distributed by and within social collectives, and it is also about how people govern relations with one another. It is about who gets what and whether the participants in (and observers of) these transactions believe them to be righteous of other kinds of human interactions–those

that seem to lie beyond material transaction and distribution. Once we understand what justice is, we can easily comprehend why it is so central to human affairs: People care deeply about how they are treated by others. (p. xv)

I define social justice as a complex interpersonal concept that evolves and changes within diverse social, cultural, historical, legal, political, and economic situations, environments, and contexts. It takes many forms, including: (1) an ideal, (2) a value or perspective, (3) a principle or standard, (4) an atmosphere or overarching climate/environment, (5) a goal or objective, (6) a process or procedure, (7) a product or policy, and (8) an end result. At the core of all forms of social justice are principles of equity, fairness, consistency, respect, and honor.

SOCIAL JUSTICE APPLICATIONS

Through the years, I have been mindful of the gap between the stated ideal and the actual implementation. Even if social justice is the purpose of an organization's existence, it is often misplaced, forgotten, and sometimes actually undermined.

In the following sections are my thoughts about how social justice should be applied. Each point is followed by specific examples. Although I am aware of experiences many others have had with regard to social justice and injustice, I reflect on just my own personal experiences in this paper.

Socially Just Environment

To achieve social justice in organizations and institutions, the climate or environment must be consistently fair, just, and ethical throughout all areas and within all components, and it must be maintained at all environmental levels, from direct practices to supervisory and managerial arenas. When consistently applied, this promotes greater stability and less organizational chaos.

In 1987, I took a leave of absence from my social work faculty position at Eastern Washington University to work as a civil rights lobbyist for the Japanese American Citizens League–Legislative Education Committee (JACL-LEC). At the time, the redress movement for Japanese Americans was in full swing. When asked to help lobby for the passage of civil rights and civil liberties legislation, I agreed and moved to Washington, D.C.

Not long after taking my new position as associate director of JACL-LEC, I was disturbed to learn that some in the organization violated the very standards and principles the organization was attempting to enforce. One administrator, for example, freely forced supervisees to work long overtime hours at night and on weekends without compensation. Employees feared that if they did not comply with the demands placed on them, they would be severely reprimanded, belittled, and fired immediately. Employees said they were further dehumanized by the boss's hostile behaviors and disparaging remarks, which they attributed to their being "non-Japanese American." Staff pointed out that the very organization that was striving for civil rights was violating the same. Consequently, I spent considerable time bringing the problem to the attention of the Board and convincing them to take corrective action (which they ultimately did).

In the same organization, I was shocked when a Board Member asked that I forge a signature on a letter that was to be sent to President Ronald Reagan. This "strategist" insisted that I sign a letter he wrote, but which was written as if it were from the sister of a heroic Japanese American soldier who was killed in action during World War II. Naturally, I refused to sign the sister's signature. Because the strategist insisted and persisted with his demand that I sign, and because it was apparent he was actually planning to send the forged letter to the President, I felt compelled to "blow the whistle." I notified other Board members in an attempt to stop this.

Both examples reveal that a socially just climate or environment can be achieved only if the participants implement and enforce social justice imperatives. These examples reveal that despite an organizational mission of social justice, equity, and fairness, its participants may be far from implementing the mission within its own organization. Some justify deviations from social justice by insisting that the ends (achieving social justice goals) justify the wrongful means (violating individual rights, manipulating the truth, and engaging in unethical and illegal behaviors). Regardless of lofty missions and goals, organizational participants must be vigilant, mindful, and action oriented.

Socially Just Processes and Interactions

One often hears the saying that, the means to achieve an end is as important as the end itself. Just processes are very important because, if unjust means are used to achieve an end, then the end is tarnished, tainted, and possibly just plain wrong. Proper and just processes should be achieved consistently and holistically.

In 2006, I was elected by the San Francisco State University School of Social Work faculty to serve as the School Director. While I was ultimately appointed to this position, the means for achieving this end left many questions about fairness and justness. After a long delay (almost an entire semester), I was finally officially appointed director by the University administration. In a nutshell, the bar for appointment was raised much higher than what was applied to others in the past. Clearly, disparate processes and procedures were at work.

After the first round of voting, I learned that I garnered the majority vote by a fraction of a vote (fractions are possible because part-time faculty votes are proportionate to their percentage teaching contract). Nevertheless, the vote results were officially announced as a "tie," thus making it necessary to vote again. I was told that in this election, one had to have a minimum of one full vote majority to win. This was very different from the standard that applied when the prior director was elected. At that time, the director was elected with only about one-third of the faculty vote–clearly far short of a majority.

In the second round of voting, I won the election with a clear majority of votes (several full votes above the majority). Although I exceeded the majority standard that was newly established for this election, I was still not appointed after the election. Yet additional steps were added. Before making the recommendation that I be appointed, the dean personally polled all tenured and tenure-track faculty and asked how they felt about my being the director. Only after he confirmed that all supported my serving as director did he submit a recommendation to SFSU's Provost and Vice President of Academic Affairs that I be appointed Chair. This process had never occurred in the history of our School. Some theorized that such disparities relate to my being a woman of color in academia.

Another example related to socially just processes is one that I experienced after I was in an automobile accident on April 15, 2007, which left me with a severe concussion, head injuries, facial cuts, spine and rib fractures, and other physical traumas and disabilities. Regardless of injuries, I returned to work about 10 days after the accident, and I was able to perform all duties associated with my usual work assignments at San Francisco State University's School of Social Work. I attended meetings, met with faculty and students, worked with students on theses and culminating projects, and carried out administrative functions related to my position as the School of Social Work's associate director and MSW Program coordinator.

Despite repeated communications and evidence to students and faculty that I was available to carry out all assignments, many imposed their own assumptions and beliefs and made decisions "for" me. In some instances, I was ignored and rendered invisible, as if incapable or non-existent. Five students in one culminating master's project began primary communications with a second reader and placed me on the copy or "cc" list, even though I was their primary sponsor. At least through his behaviors and actions, the professor who was the second reader promoted such behavior even after I communicated my objections. After meeting with this professor, one of my student advisees dubbed him as "advisor standing in for Rita Takahashi."

In an e-mail message to some faculty, I responded to their query as to what was going on with regard to issues of my disability. I identified many of the same forms of disparate, insensitive, and discriminatory treatment as one experiences as a person of color. Because some faculty did not seem "to get it," I explicitly stated (in an e-mail message) what I assessed was going on, and I connected the social work skills we are supposed to be teaching:

> Here are a few of the many social work skills involved in what has transpired [after I was injured in the car accident]: (1) Ask or check it out before jumping to conclusion(s). (2) Check assumptions, and conduct the faulty assumption test. (3) Do one's homework and check facts before taking action. (4) Be mindful that, while one might have good intentions, the result might be paternalistic.(5) Be sensitive to cross cultural differences and diverse interpretations and spin. (6) Collaborate before "deciding or speaking for." (7) Know and understand how one contributes to oppression of others via multiple means. (8) Check one's conclusions for value and belief projections, which may not apply in other cultural contexts. (9) Think about what one's proper role and function should be, given the situation and context. (10) Check, apply, and assess multiple forms of social justice: from interactional to process justice.

Socially Just Interactions and Treatment

To achieve socially just interactions, persons in organizations and institutions must be treated fairly and equitably. Communications should be collaborative and cooperative. Participants must have equal access to information and within the same or similar time frames.

In organizations, I have experienced multiple forms of inequities and disparities. In some situations, a person who is aligned or identified with a person in power gets exclusive and timely communications and information needed to competitively vie for resources, including grants, stipends, and perks. This places others at an unfair or nonexistent position for equitable resources.

Interactions that are positive, collegial, and respectful are important to achieving social justice. Unfortunately, this is has not been achieved in many organizations and institutions. According to Sue et al. (2007),

> Although the civil rights movement had a significant effect on changing racial interactions in this society, racism continues to plague the United States (p. 271).

Through the years, I have seen and experienced various forms of racial microaggressions, which Sue et al. (2007) define as:

> . . . brief and commonplace daily verbal, behavioral, and environmental indignities, whether intentional or unintentional, that communicate hostile, derogatory, or negative racial slights and insults to the target person or group. They are not limited to human encounters alone but may also be environmental in nature, as when a person of color is exposed to an office setting that unintentionally assails his or her racial identity. . . . Three forms of microaggressions can be identified: microassault, microinsult, and microinvalidation. (pp. 273-274)

All who are outside the dominant culture group are affected by microaggressions when dominant standards, values, and modes of operation are imposed. The dynamics and impact are often submerged or invisible. Thus, Sue et al. (2007) submit that "the greatest challenge society and the mental health professions face is making the 'invisible' 'visible'" (p. 281).

Socially Just Policies and Procedures

Consistent and equitable applications of policies and procedures are important. In the United States, rule of law, policies, and procedures are utilized as guides and mandates for behaviors. Established policies and procedures are only as good as they are instituted, applied, and enforced.

In reality, there are many inconsistencies and gaps. One example I experienced related to compensation for work. The current general rule at San Francisco State University is that faculty may not get paid an overload, and they cannot get additional salary for administering a School or University contract if they are already receiving full salary. This would be fine, except that this rule has been inconsistently applied. As the incoming new director of the School, I became the principal investigator for several projects; yet I will receive no additional salary. Rather, allocated funds for the principal investigator will go into the School's pool of resources. This was not the case for the prior White director, as she received additional salary throughout her tenure as director. In fact, she continued to be paid through the last month of her active employment as director. Immediately after she left, I became the director and assumed all principal investigator duties the previous director had, but I received none of the additional salary compensation she garnered for years.

Another inconsistency that I experienced involved the processes and procedures used for director appointment. The procedure for electing the school director dramatically changed this year. In prior years, faculty simply placed their names on a ballot, and if they opted to do so, they wrote a statement. In the recent election, director candidates were asked to write a position and action statement, and they had to appear before the faculty and staff to present statements and field questions. At a second meeting, the candidates debated each other before the School (faculty, staff and students).

An additional example in which policies or procedures varied involved office space. When I became the Bachelor of Arts in Social Work (BASW) coordinator, I was promised an unshared office to myself, just as the prior White BASW coordinator had for years when she was the director. This never transpired, and the perks were inconsistently applied. While the BASW Coordinator, I always had to share an office with at least one additional faculty person.

Socially Just Products and Results

An important form of social justice is realized through results and end products. For fairness, persons should have equitable access and opportunities to compete and achieve desired ends.

Inequitable and unjust results are apparent in many organizations and institutions. Despite being situated in highly diverse areas, many institutions fall short of reflecting the diversity of the communities surrounding them. Lack of diverse representativeness (by class, ethnic/cultural background, gender, age, physical ability, sexual orientation, and more) is especially apparent in higher levels of management and administration.

In many of life's arenas, equity simply does not prevail. Studies reveal how persons are subjected to discrimination on the individual, group, and macro societal levels. This, according to Gilbert Gee et al. (2007), affects not only the person's standing in life, but also the person's health. In a national Latino and Asian American study reported in the May and July 2007 issues of the *American Journal of Public Health,* researchers found that discrimination and stress stemming from such discrimination are associated with multiple health problems, including cardiovascular and respiratory conditions, substance use, and chronic illnesses. Mozes (2007) quotes authors of this article, saying that "race still matters," and adding:

> So what's important is that we keep acknowledging that discrimination does occur and find ways to combat it as well as to continue policies that promote civil rights.

In organizations, I have seen what I believe are multiple forms of discrimination, but they are often difficult to prove. The impact, however, is very clear. All forms of microaggressions (Sue et al., 2007) impinge on one's overall health, welfare, and happiness. Further, they can have longer-term impact on subsequent generations, because historical trauma becomes an embedded and multi-generational experience (Takahashi, 2001).

Needed Actions

Social workers and the social work profession have expressed support for social justice, but much must be done to reveal a solid commitment and to achieve substantial results. We must go beyond talking about social justice and articulating it as a mission or goal. We need to define what we mean, understand and articulate its many forms, establish ways to implement and maintain all aspects of social justice, analyze results, evaluate/assess results, and retool or change for positive results.

REFERENCES

Folger, R. & Cropanzano, R. (1998). *Organizational justice and human resource management.* Thousand Oaks, CA: Sage Publications.

Gee, G. C., Spencer, M. S., Chen, J., & Takeuchi, D. (2007, July). A nationwide study of discrimination and chronic health conditions among Asian Americans. *American Journal of Public Health,* 97 (7), pp. 1275-1282.

Mozes, Alan. (2007, May 31). *Health Day News.* Available at: http://aast.wordpress.com/ 2007/07/01/discrimination-linked-to-chronic-health-problems-for-asian-americans/. Accessed July 17, 2007.

Sue, D. W., Capodilupo, C. M., Torino, G. C., Bucceri, J. M., Holder, A. M. B., Nadal, K. L., & Esquilin, M. (2007, May-June). Racial microaggressions in everyday life: Implications for clinical practice. *American Psychologist,* 62 (4), pp. 271-286.

Takahashi, R. (2004). "Japanese Americans and the historical trauma of exclusion and incarceration." Unpublished manuscript submitted to Maria Yellow Horse Brave Heart for publication in her edited book on historical trauma.

Mexican Migration for Dummies: What Social Workers and the Public Need to Know

Kurt C. Organista

INTRODUCTION

The title of this article is not intended to insult the reader, but rather to convey how very simple the basic dynamics of Mexican migration to the United States really are. Yet the root causes of undocumented migration are sorely missing from the current derisive debate about *border control, national security,* and *"illegal aliens"* that has inspired the organization of self-proclaimed "vigilance" citizen groups such as the Minutemen, and ironically has also motivated millions of Mexican workers and immigrants, undocumented and documented alike, to organize themselves at the grassroots level to refute this latest wave of anti-immigrant, anti-Mexican rhetoric at the highest levels of government.

Such rhetoric continues to fuel immigration policies that are ultimately detrimental to the economic security of both the U.S. and Mexico, certainly to Mexican and American workers, and to the very lives of migrants crossing an increasingly dangerous border that has claimed well over 2,000 lives since 1993, or between 150 and 200 lives per year on average. Besides, the American public has grown to love and rely on that endearing line of books by the same title!

The interesting thing about vital information on Mexican migration is that it has been well documented for decades by dozens of prominent social scientists applying multiple explanatory theories, backed up by large scale research projects (e.g., The Mexican Migration Project by Douglas Massey and colleagues). Nevertheless, this important reservoir of information is rarely if ever tapped by politicians, public leaders, or even migrants and their advocates, too many of whom debate the issue with shallow hyperbole. We simply must get past superficial level arguments on both sides as reflected in overused statements such as, "They broke the law by crossing over illegally and should be jailed and deported" on the one hand, and on the other, "I'm not a criminal because I work, pay taxes, and help the United States."

Social workers or *anyone* assisting undocumented migrants, including teachers, health care providers, clergy and parishioners, need a firm grasp on the historical and current facts of Mexican migration, especially considering multiple recent congressional bills. Examples include the bill introduced on December 6, 2005, by Senator James Sensenbrenner of Wisconsin (ironically a historical farm state that relied considerably on

Mexican farm workers), and the one eventually passed by the House of Representatives 10 days later (the so-called Border Protection Anti-Terror and Illegal Immigration Control Act of 2005), advocating that it be made a *felony* for anyone to provide assistance to undocumented people in need. When you consider that a felony is a high crime that includes things like rape and murder, it makes sense that such bills are being called "absurd" by the Mexican President Felipe Calderon (Roig-Franzia, 2007) a human rights violation by the Catholic Church, and why the NASW advocates "replacing the current patchwork of immigration laws and procedures with a fair, equitable and comprehensive national plan" (NASW, 2006). Should social workers follow the lead of the Catholic Church in asserting that they will continue to serve immigrants in need regardless of which bills are eventually enforced? The migration-related orientation and arguments below will help support this moral position. Social and human service providers know better than anyone that there is no clear line between documented and undocumented people given that both statuses populate the same families and communities.

A grounded understanding of Mexican migration begins with being informed about three important and overlapping areas: (1) The historically strained state of U.S.-Mexico relations; (2) the historical pattern of Mexican labor use and abuse, and (3) the integration of the economies of the U.S. and Mexico, as formalized by NAFTA, into one major inter-locking global economic system that creates a *migration bridge* for the undocumented as a bi-product.

A BRIEF HISTORICAL ANALYSIS OF MEXICAN MIGRATION TO THE U.S.

Strained U.S.-Mexico Relations

The old Mexican saying, *México, tan lejos de dios y tan cerca de los Estados Unidos* [Mexico, so far from god and so close to the United States], emerges from 150 years of strained relations between these two nations rooted in international war, major loss of land holdings following the defeat of Mexico, and *continuous* exploitation of Mexican labor. The labor supplied by millions of Mexican labor migrants is essential to billion dollar American corporations, industries, and work sectors such as agricultural farm work, fishing and forestry jobs, day labor, construction, landscaping and gardening, meat packing and poultry production, domestic cleaning, child and elderly care, hotel and office building janitorial services, and the vast and expanding service sector.

Best estimates by the D.C.-based Urban Institute of Immigration Studies count over 9 million undocumented immigrants in the U.S., 80% of whom are Latino, two-thirds of whom are employed, thus constituting 5% of the entire U.S. workforce. The idea of criminalizing 5% of the American workforce not only seems far fetched, but it would be a significant threat to the economy if such workers were arrested and deported. It's worth noting here that in response to the inflammatory arguments of politicians and citizen groups claiming that the undocumented are an economic "drain" on public services, social workers and other advocates should ask them why they fail to mention the nearly $200 billion dollars in unclaimed social security taxes steadily accruing in the U.S. treasury (Downes, 2006). They should also remind them that 500 leading U.S. economists, including 5 Nobel Prize winners, argue in their "Open Letter to President Bush and Congress" that not only is immigration a net economic gain for the U.S. and its citizens, but it is also the "greatest anti-poverty program ever devised" (Theroux, 2006).

The increasingly popular new saying that "People don't cross borders, borders cross people" could have been coined by the estimated 75,000 to 100,000 Mexicans who instantly became American citizens by default (minus property protection) when Mexico lost the war with the U.S. in the mid-1800s, an eventuality that grew out of the Battle of the Alamo in 1836 when American settlers claimed Mexican land as their own independent "Republic of Texas" and faced the predictable consequences. Mexico had provided free land to hundreds of thousands of Westward expansion settlers on the condition that they obey Mexican law and apply for Mexican citizenship. While some settlers complied, most did not and crossed into Mexico illegally, an ironic historical footnote given today's indignant finger pointing at undocumented Mexicans.

Mexico's defeat included being coerced to surrender about half of its land or the present day Southwest. Mexican inhabitants of this territory became, in effect, the first Mexican laborers in the U.S. when devious schemes were used to dispossess them of their land. For example, Mexican inhabitants were charged property taxes they were unable to pay leading to land seizures and sales to American settlers who were then charged lower taxes. Mexico's lingering resentment was symbolized by the use of maps in Mexican schools, through the 1940s, that designated Northern Mexico as "territory temporarily in the hands of the United States." (McWilliams, 1968, p. 103).

Decade by Decade Analysis of Mexican Labor Migration During the 20th Century

Evident below is a cyclical pattern of exploiting poor Mexican workers during labor shortages followed by abusing their human and civil rights during economic recessions:

1910s. During the World War I labor shortage in agriculture, about 70,000 Mexicans were allowed to enter the U.S. to perform farmwork when U.S. federal authorities waived immigration restrictions for Mexico. The violent decade of the Mexican revolution (1910 to 1920) also pushed these labor migrants and other Mexicans to *El Norte.*

1920s. New markets opened during the 1920s with improved canning and shipping technologies luring approximately a half million Mexicans with little if any regard for their documentation status. Also, while The Immigration Act of 1924 barred the majority of southern and eastern Europeans from immigrating to the U.S., Mexico was again exempted, because it had become the main source of cheap labor to major industries such as mining, railroads and, of course, agriculture, essential to the development of the Southwestern U.S.

1930s. But when the Great Depression struck in 1929, Congress decided to make undocumented immigration to the U.S. a felony and authorized massive deportation campaigns against Mexicans who were scapegoated for country's economic problems. An estimated 500,000 or 40% of the Mexican American population were either deported or coerced to leave in a program called Repatriation, often regardless of documentation status.

1940s. Despite the abuse of Mexican labor migrants in the previous decade, when the World War II labor shortage occurred in 1942, the U.S. quickly initiated a bi-national agreement with Mexico to import agricultural labor. The Bracero Program brought in an estimated 5 million *Braceros* to work the fields from 1942 to 1964 (*Bracero* is from the word *brazo* or "arm," a loose translation of "work hand"). Predictably, the Bracero program also stimulated a parallel stream of undocumented workers especially desirable to employers preferring to avoid the Bracero Program's bureaucratic procedures that included stipulations of fair pay and treatment of Mexican workers.

1950s. National level fear of communists during the McCarthy era led to border control in the name of national security and the initiation in 1954 of a program with the derogatory title "Operation Wetback," that resulted in the deportation of about 80,000 Mexicans, and 10 times as many Mexicans fleeing to Mexico to avoid apprehension. The civil rights of Mexican Americans were frequently violated as homes and businesses were raided for suspected "illegal aliens." Interestingly, during this same period, upwards of a million deported Mexicans were delivered not to the IRS, but to the Department of Labor that quickly processed them as Braceros and promptly returned them to the very farms from which they were deported. Both growers and a hoodwinked public were pleased.

1960s and 1970s. The Bracero program was halted by Mexico in 1964, because of the mistreatment of Mexican laborers in Texas, the same year that strict immigration quotas were extended to Mexico for the very first time (only 120,000 per year). The predictable result of this restrictive immigration policy was an unprecedented surge in undocumented Mexican labor migration, lasting 20 years, due to the expanding need for cheap labor in the U.S. combined with a lack of consequences for employers hiring undocumented workers. In effect, what was created during this era was an informal Bracero Program. Today a mere 5,000 visas are available each year to unskilled Mexican laborers, not only a number sorely out of touch with demand, but guaranteed to reinforce undocumented migration.

1980s. Unexpectedly, the discovery of vast oil reserves in Mexico quickly lead to bankruptcy when the country over-invested in oil infrastructure that failed to pay off when the price of oil plummeted on the international market. Mexico's economic collapse was called the "lost decade," and it accelerated out-migration to the U.S. Not able to pay its foreign debt to the U.S., with no offer of loan forgiveness, a desperate Mexico had little choice but to give in to U.S. demands to lift trade taxes and tariffs, paving the way for free trade. Meanwhile, the U.S. passed the Immigration Reform and Control Act (IRCA) of 1986 that granted amnesty to nearly 2 million undocumented migrants that had accrued since 1964. IRCA also authorized major fines and penalties for *knowingly* hiring the undocumented. Not surprisingly, this new hiring law was never enforced, partly because of the rise of false documents. Newly legalized farmworkers quickly deserted the fields in search of better jobs and were immediately replaced by labor migrants comprised of more undocumented than ever before (today most farmworkers are undocumented).

1990s. During the last decade of the 20th century, the integration of U.S. and Mexican economies was formalized with the signing of the North American Free Trade Agreement (NAFTA) on New Year's Day, 1994. Ironically, this was the same year in which restrictions on immigration reached new heights with "Operation Gatekeeper" or the militarization of the border that included erecting a 14 mile long steel fence in California. More recently in May of 2006, the Senate backed a bill authorizing 370 miles of triple fencing along the entire border at a cost of 3.2 million per mile. But the glaring problem with an "open border" policy for trade and a "closed border" policy for immigration is that you simply cannot have it both ways for reasons explained below.

HOW THE U.S. CREATES UNDOCUMENTED MEXICAN LABOR MIGRATION

Severely restrictive immigration policies cannot coexist with NAFTA-styled free trade without creating an undocumented *migration bridge* for three simple reasons:

1. By design, NAFTA has increased U.S.-Mexico trade tenfold since it began, and thus increased the number of business-related border crossings, as well as a parallel stream of undocumented crossings in the process. Think about 10 times as many border crossings by business visitors, inter-company transfers, contract and temporary workers; 10 times as many automobiles, trucks, trains, planes, and boats transporting goods, and good old-fashioned foot traffic, and then ask yourself if a similar increase in undocumented crossings is also likely to co-occur. If the answer is yes (and it is by the way) then such predictable shadow crossings must be anticipated and properly managed.

2. While NAFTA has significantly increased trade for both countries, it has also displaced hundreds of thousands of workers in both urban and rural Mexico. For example, to attract U.S. investors, NAFTA reforms required the privatization of factories, railroads, airlines, and other government-owned businesses, resulting in waves of layoffs. Meanwhile in rural Mexico, subsistence farmers, small businesses, artisans, and laborers are increasingly displaced by the mechanization of local agriculture by U.S. businesses, self-eliminating competition between small farmers to supply American businesses with cash crops, and the importation of U.S. goods and services with which local business simply cannot compete.

Further, the American product assembly or *maquiladora* industry, with over 2,000 plants just south of the border, has feminized local workforces in Northern Mexico with poverty wages for women and no work for men. Unfortunately under NAFTA, breaking maquiladora strikes and unions on the border has become an essential part of what is called the Border Industrialization Program. According to the Mexican

Migration Project, unprecedented U.S. expansion into Mexican land, raw materials, local markets, and labor exacerbates regional economic instability, produces significant unemployment, and thus out-migration to the U.S. It should also be noted that between 500,000 and a million U.S. jobs have been lost to the *maquiladora* industry and that low SES American workers have trouble competing with undocumented workers, employed in order to keep wages depressed at the bottom of the pay scale.

3. NAFTA's explicit focus on the movement of *capital* and not the movement of *labor* automatically advantages the U.S. and disadvantages Mexico when you consider the surpluses each country has to offer. But why can't NAFTA be revised to also focus on the movement of labor, including worker's rights, considering continued U.S. dependence on Mexican labor in our expanding service sector economy? Thus, herein lies the 3rd reason for unabated undocumented labor migration to the United States: Mexican labor is not only pushed by NAFTA dynamics and Mexico's economic instability, but also continues to be powerfully pulled by the increasing demand for cheap unskilled and semi-skilled labor in America's vast and growing service sector, as well as other cheap labor dependent business sectors. As the comedian and political satirist Bill Mauer recently joked, if you really wanted to decrease undocumented migration, you'd give American workers a real living wage.

LATINO LABOR MIGRATION IN THE 21ST CENTURY

Bridges to Economic and Social Development in the Western Hemispheric or Undocumented Labor?

So why not develop sensible, non-contradictory immigration and economic policies, sensitive to the different needs, resources, and *social* development of each country, including the regulation of Mexican labor migration to the U.S. given its vital role in the formally integrated economies of the U.S. and Mexico? Thirteen years in the making, it appears that NAFTA has not delivered on it's promise to decrease Mexican labor migration by helping Mexico become economically independent (as opposed to dependent on U.S. goods, services, and cheap wages). In fact, Mexico has become economically dependent on the remittances of labor migrants in the U.S., who sent back 23 billion *migra-dollars* in 2006 according to estimates by the Mexican government based on *Banco de México* databases of monthly transfers. Surely such remittances underscore the need for NAFTA to also focus on the movement of Mexican labor in addition to capital between these major trading partners.

Thus, now is the time to oppose the contradiction of restrictive immigration and permissive global economic policies that produce undocumented migration bridges, especially in view of the Bush administration's current plans to extend NAFTA to Central and South America by establishing FTAA or Free Trade Area of the Americas. It is probably a good sign that when President Bush met with Latin American trade ministers in Miami in November of 2003, that those from Brazil, Argentina, Venezuela, and Ecuador rejected the plan in view of the Mexican example. However, the example of Mexico also demonstrates how easily poor countries indebted to the U.S. can be coerced to sign on to free trade American-style.

Rather than continuing to construct millions of legally and socially marginalized undocumented workers, vulnerable to labor exploitation, human rights violations, and public scorn, and threatening professionals and citizens with prison for providing humanitarian assistance to them, the U.S. must own up to its responsibility for this important population that it shares in common with Mexico. Any seductive short-term economic advantages of the current contradictory system are not worth the long-term consequence of having economically and socially unstable and U.S.- dependent neighbors throughout Latin America. U.S.-Mexico migration scholar Susan Sassen (1990) eloquently expressed this very assertion more than a decade and a half ago:

> The implications for the Mexican case are clear. Migrations are produced. The mere fact of a shared border and inequality in wages between the two countries is not sufficient in itself to account for immigration. The construction of railroads in the 1800s, the development of commercial agriculture, and now the development of the Border Industrialization Program are all processes which created a labor market. The fact that this labor market was eventually divided by a patrolled border led to contradictions in the legislation covering both halves. Secondly, if the United States, through it's economic activities, has incorporated Mexican workers and Mexican areas into a broader international organization of production, and if, furthermore, these activities promote the formation of migrations, then the United States must assume some responsibility for immigration of Mexicans into North America.

REFERENCES

Downes, L. (2006). Talking points: The terrible, horrible, urgent national disaster that immigration isn't. *New York Times*, June 20, 2006.

McWilliams, C. (1968). *North from Mexico: The Spanish-Speaking People of the United States*. New York: Greenwood Press, Publishers.

NASW (2006). Border Protection Anti-Terrorism and Illegal Immigration and Control Act of 2005. Government Relations Update. https://www.socialworkers.org/advocacy/updates/2006/032406.asp

Roig-Franzia, M. (2007). Mexican president criticizes 'absurd' U.S. border policies. *Washington Post*, March 17, A10.

Sassen, S. (1990). Immigration policy towards Mexico in a global economy. *Journal of International Affairs, 43*(2), 369-383.

Theroux, D. (2006). Open letter on immigration. Washington, D.C.: The Independent Institute.

Marches on Washington
and the Black Protest Movement

Charles Green
Basil Wilson

INTRODUCTION

Between 1995 and 2005, a series of million marches have been held by Black community leaders. In October 1995, a march called by Minister Louis Farrakhan, the leader of the Nation of Islam, attracted an enormous gathering of Black men at the capital Mall in Washington, D.C. But the call for the March was deemed controversial and conventional politicians, White and Black, mainstream media, and even the President of the United States denounced Farrakhan as a hatemonger.

There was much discussion in the Black community and in the mainstream media about the gender bias of the March. Black feminists denounced the March as an expression of the persistence of patriarchy in the Black community. Despite the mainstream efforts to negate the event, the Million Man March captured the imagination of a multi-generation of Black men who assembled in the U.S. capital by the tens of thousands. Whether a million marchers assembled or a half million, everyone agreed that it was a massive turning out of what some consider to be an endangered species.

In October 1997, a group of grassroots women held a Million Woman March in Philadelphia. Again, the turnout of Black women was enormous. Much of the organization of the Million Woman March was done on the Internet. The keynote speaker was Winnie Mandela, the former wife of the iconoclastic South African Prime Minister, Nelson Mandela. For certain, The Million Woman March and the Million Man March that preceded it struck a chord in the Black community, and the throngs who attended were reflecting a new sense of political anxiety.

Over the Labor Day weekend of September 1998, two separate Million Youth Marches were called, one for New York City and the other in Atlanta, Georgia. The Atlanta Youth March included a coalition of the Nation of Islam, Operation PUSH, and the NAACP. Nonetheless, the March failed to attract the massive numbers seen at the Washington and Philadelphia marches.

The Million Youth March suffered a similar fate in New York City. This march which was staged in Harlem, was called by the late Khallid Muhammad, a former spokesman for the Nation of Islam, who became renown for his anti-semitic rhetoric. Moreover, the court struggles surrounding the march made it impossible to predict if permission to hold the march would have been given. Muhammad did receive some support from Black nationalist circles in New York City, but the siege mentality surrounding the march ensured that the turnout would be a far cry from the numbers achieved in Washington, D.C. and in Philadelphia.

The Republican Administration at City Hall vehemently opposed the staging of a march in Harlem and refused to grant permission for the march. Once the court permission was granted at the eleventh hour, Mayor Giuliani begrudgingly consented. He ensured that the designated areas for the march were "corralled" off by police barriers and that subway routes leading directly to the march were disrupted. There were as many police as there were marchers. The march permit specified that it had to conclude by four o'clock, and a few minutes before the hour, police helicopters swooped down on the protest crowd and the riot unit of the New York Police Department moved in to disperse the crowd.

This chapter seeks to examine a mass march phenomenon in the African American community. What are the issues precipitating this ethos of anxiety in Black civil society that has found expression in the call for million marches? The chapter will compare the Civil Rights Movement with the million march events. The chapter concludes with an assessment of why this mass assembly of Black people has failed to sustain itself and to become a potent political force in American society.

THE POST-CIVIL RIGHTS ANXIETY

Politics in America has always been profoundly affected by the state racial dialectics. Whether one begins with the issue of slavery in America, the Abolitionist Movement, the Civil War, Reconstruction or the Post-Reconstruction years of Jim Crow, the racial dialectic appears at the epicenter of American politics. The gains of the Civil Rights Movement were instrumental in bringing the Black community into the conventional political equation. At that juncture, the South was desegregated and the Black voter and Black elected officials became an integral part of the political landscape. There are presently over 40 Black elected Congressional representatives, and where the Black community is unduly concentrated, Black elected officials exercise some power in state and city politics. But the presence of Black elected officials is largely visible in the Democratic Party, and this has triggered a regional and racial realignment of party politics in contemporary America. In the post-Civil War period, the Democratic Party in the South accommodated itself to racists of every stripe. Blacks identified with the party of Lincoln and voted for Republican candidates. The converse has taken place in the post-civil rights years. Whites have shifted their political allegiance to the Republican Party and the Republican Party in the South and elsewhere has become the refuge of what remains of the racist forces in America.

When Kevin Phillips wrote *The Emerging Republican Majority* in 1968, he identified certain changing demographics in American society with the population shift taking place in the West and Southwest areas of the country that were more conservative than the liberal Northeast. Phillips helped to perpetuate the myth that Blacks were able to exercise undue influence in the Democratic Party and thus many White Democrats were alienated from the party and gravitated to the Republican Party. Beginning in the 1980s with the election of Ronald Reagan to the Presidency, there were signs that Republican hegemony could emerge and be in a position to assert conservative domination over the judicial, executive, and congressional branches of government.

Beginning with the election of Franklin Delano Roosevelt to the Presidency in 1932, political scientists have designated the years of 1932-68 as years in which liberal thought and the Democratic party prevailed for forty years, despite the two terms of President Eisenhower from 1952-60. Although Reagan won the Presidency in the 1980s, the Democrats had control of the House and for the most part the Senate. It was only in 1994 that the Republican Party began to take control of the House of Representatives and the Senate. Under the leadership of speaker Newt Gingrich, the Republicans embarked on an aggressive policy of rolling back benefits gained by the Black population, such as welfare entitlements and affirmative action.

It certainly is not happenstance that one year after the Republicans took control of the House of Representatives, there was a call for the Million Man March. But the ethos of anxiety felt by Blacks was not confined to the politics of the capital. Even liberal states like New York had moved demonstrably to the right. Racist elements, sometimes distinguishable, oftentimes not from the conservative tide, became more politically strident in matters affecting the Black community.

What is triggering this racial animus? Much of the present racial animus can be traced to the conservative opposition to legislation passed during the height of the Civil Rights Movement and the presumption that such legislation is injurious to the well-being of American civilization. In the same year that Congress passed the Voting Rights Act, Congress passed the 1965 Immigration Bill that eliminated racial preference from entry into the United States. This change in the immigration law has changed and made more complex the racial dialectic in America. America in the twenty-first century has become a cultural society. After thirty years of an immigration law that transcended race and ethnicity,

America has become a multi-racial, multi-cultural nation particularly in the coastal states in the West, Southwest and Northeast.

New racist groups like the Council of Conservative Citizens and American Renaissance are troubled by the state of diminished whiteness in America. At the 1998 American Renaissance Conference held in Northern Virginia, syndicated columnist, Samuel Francis, noted that "the Founders and most of the great men of the past clearly intended the United States to be a white nation" (James Luneskas, 1998). Much of this sentiment could be depicted in the national debate inside and outside of Congress with the failure to deal with the plight of 12 million undocumented aliens.

There are other events and policies that have given rise to this White ethos of anxiety. Sizeable segments of the White community have been effectively marginalized by globalization. The Black community was terribly impacted by the deindustrialization that made the position of Black labor beginning in the 1970s superfluous. The position of the Black community has increased in class variegation, and the state in recent decades has become more and more praetorian.

Passage of welfare legislation in the 1930s was a way of accommodating capitalist society to the fact that it was unable to maintain high levels of employment during periods of economic contraction and even in periods of economic expansion. Republicans and centrist Democrats alike have embraced a more punitive version of the welfare state, one that appears less magnanimous and more brutish.

Another sense of anxiety in the Black community comes from the massive expansion of the penal system. America is now a society of penal colonies comprised of a disproportionate number of Black male youths. African Americans constitute 13 percent of the population, yet approximately fifty percent of the prison population. The prison population has been increasing exponentially, and the war on drugs pursued by the federal government and "broken windows" strategies pursued by police departments on the state level have hardened the nature of the American criminal justice system. For example, in New York State prisons, there were 24,000 inmates in 1980 and by 1990, there were approximately 70,000. The new criminal justice aggressiveness from policing to mandatory sentencing occurred at a juncture when the capitalist system in America became less consensual and more coercive. The attack on the World Trade Center and on the Pentagon have made the American state terrified of forces inside and outside of America.

BLACK LEGISLATORS AND THE CONSERVATIVE TIDE

Black elected officials tend to be concentrated on the liberal spectrum of the Democratic Party. Since the Clinton era of the 1990s, that liberal spectrum has become a minority in the party as the majority of White Democrats have moved to the center and have become indistinguishable from the Republican right in matters of criminal justice policy, welfare-to work programs, and the minimization of the state in the lives of working people. Since the Democratic Party took back control of Congress in 2006, there have been some shifts from the center and a greater commitment to health care, raising minimum wages, and raising higher education assistance.

In the New York State legislature and in the City Council, there exist Black and Latino caucuses. Decision making in these bodies are highly centralized around the Speaker of the Assembly or the Majority leader of the City Council. These caucuses invariably support the party leadership and have not been able to temper some of the more draconian legislation having to do with the criminal justice system, the welfare system or even in the inadequate funding for public and higher education.

The leadership of the mass march events has come from Black nationalist forces rather than from Black elected officials. Playing the vanguard role have been members of the Nation of Islam. Because of the publicity and successful mobilization surrounding the Million Man March, many elected and unelected officials like Harlem's senior Congressman Charles Rangel and Rev. Jesse Jackson were willing to speak at the 1995 and 2005 marches. But the 1995 and 2005 marches were essentially a show put on by the Nation of Islam.

The Million Women March in Philadelphia was not initially controlled by the Nation of Islam, but as the event mushroomed, the role of the Nation of Islam in providing security became more salient. The Million Youth March in New York City which sputtered had as the driving force an exiled spokesperson of the Nation of Islam. Among the various nationalist leaders in New York City who spoke from the platform were Conrad Muhammad, formerly the Minister of the Mosque Number 7 in Harlem and now the self-designated Minister for the Hip Hop generation, Elombe Brathe of the December 12 Movement, and Rev. Al Sharpton of the African National Network. Presently, the Black nationalist leadership represents a resistance against racism.

There have been some attempts to define the movement through the agreed upon mission statement adopted for the Million Man March. Written and presented at the march by Maulana Karenga, the march's mission statement is a progressive document. Karenga makes reference to the inclusive nature of the document and that it constitutes the outgrowth of the over 318 local organizing committees.

Prior to the march in 1995, a National Organizing Committee was established that reflected the different schools of thought that came under the umbrella of the Million Man March. Karenga reflects the ethos of anxiety in the Black community when he writes of "profound concern for increasing racism, deteriorating social and environmental conditions and the urgent need for transformation and progressive leadership in such a context" (Karenga, 1995). Concern about the right wing Republican hegemony of Congress in 1994 is presented in the document:

> Recognizing that the country and government have made a dangerous and regressive turn to the right and are producing policies with negative impact on people of color, the poor, and the vulnerable . . . (Karenga, 1995).

The collective mission statement indicted the United States government for the criminal justice policies that have been operationalized over the last two decades:

> We call on the government to also atone for its role in criminalizing a whole people, for its policies of destroying, discrediting, disrupting and otherwise neutralizing Black leadership, for spending more money on imprisonment than education, and on weapons of war than social development, for dismantling regulations that restrained corporations in their degradation of the environment and failing to check a deadly environmental racism that encourages placement of a toxic waste in communities of color. (Karenga 1995)

The Million Man March on Washington focused not only on the external environment, but sought to bring about behavioral changes within the Black community. Three themes that defined the March were: atonement, reconciliation, and responsibility. There was some concern by left-oriented Black intellectuals like Horace Campbell (1997) who felt the emphasis on atonement played into the hands of White conservatives and ended up blaming the victim. But it was the mystic nature of Farrakhan's closing address that helped to underscore the conservative message of the march. As Karenga noted:

> After the spiritual cleansing of atonement, it was necessary to take personal and collective responsibility for our lives and the welfare and future of our families and our community. (Karenga, 1995)

Despite the conservative tendency in certain parts of the mission statement, the document reaffirmed the tradition of Black resistance to racism and the necessity to struggle for the just society. The mission statement reflects the variegated nature of nationalist and progressive schools of thought that came together to dramatize the Black condition in contemporary America.

The Million More March held ten years after the Million Man March on October 15, 2005 was also held in the capital, Washington, D.C., but in ten years the United States found itself in a different relationship to the rest of the world. The Cold War had ended, but the United States was embroiled in an Armageddon war against the forces of terrorism. As far as the Washington decision-makers were concerned, as of 9/11, 2001, the world had changed. The Black condition or the racial dialectic was not what was critical, rather the threat that Al Queda presented at home and abroad.

The Million More March brought together Black organizations of all stripes. Farrakhan was instrumental in forging this unity. The March outlined ten burning issues for the Black community: (1) unity; (2) spiritual values; (3) education; (4) economic development; (5) political power; (6) reparations; (7) denunciation of the prison industrial complex; (8) the need for informal health care; (9) the responsibility of the White to the Black community; (10) the critical nature of peace in the world and in the Black community.

Minister Louis Farrakhan addressed many of these issues in his closing address. Farrakhan denounced the aggressive behavior of United States foreign policy in the Middle East and denounced the deception that led us into war with Iraq. The leader of the Nation of Islam, who had developed a reputation for intolerance, made a case for religious tolerance and peace in the world.

DEFINING A MOVEMENT

Despite the unity of the Million More March, the quest for movement has not been able to sustain much of a momentum. Nothing of any import has crystallized in the Black community and after the 2005 march, the local organizing committees melted into a state of invisibility. The quintessential question to arise, therefore, is whether we can accurately define the million marches as a movement or non-movement?

Sociologists of collective behavior and social movements distinguish between true social movements and riots, panics, crazes, and other forms of crowd action. The literature reflects the debate that has ensued around this distinction and too the effect of mass action on the social system. Earlier theorists including Le Bon were critical of what was termed crowd action. Participants were cast off as blind followers, "mindless masses," or as if part of a herd. Kornhauser (1959), Lipset (1959), and Smelser (1962) all investigate the deficiencies in society that prove conducive to the growth of mass action. Alienation according to Kornhauser heightens responsiveness to the appeal of mass movements, because they provide occasions for expressing resentment against what is, as well as the promise of a totally different world. Whereas collective behavior refers to a continuum of non-routine behaviors that are engaged in by large numbers of people, social movements are forms of collective behavior that represent intentional efforts by groups in a society to create new institutions or to reform existing ones (Kornblum, 1997; Goldberg, 1991). Social movements can take different forms depending upon the ideological trajectory of their leaders and followers. There are reactionary movements and conservative movements as well as reformist movements and revolutionary movements.

In *Black Movements in America*, Cedric Robinson considers this ideological torrent in the Black community. He notes that for nearly 400 years Black Americans have been torn between two constructions of America, the Jeffersonian promise of a just republic and the nightmare of racial oppression. Based on his examination of the historical records of slave resistance movements in the U.S. from the sixteenth and seventeenth centuries to the civil rights movements, Robinson argues that Blacks have constructed both a culture of resistance and a culture of accommodation based on the radically different experiences of slaves and free Blacks. He concludes that contemporary Black movements are inspired by either a social vision–held by the relatively privileged strata or that of the masses–which interprets the Black experience in America as proof of the country's hypocrisy (Robinson, 1994). While some like Robinson give support to radical movements for change in the African American community, other Black scholars and activists are inspired by reformist and conventionalist approaches. To the untrained observer, the question whether a specific collective activity suggests a social movement might seem trivial or perhaps a meaningless exercise on the part of scholars. However, to persons committed to bringing about constructive social change, this is seen as extremely critical.

In their seminal study on poor people's movements, Piven and Cloward (1979) underscore the importance of positive leadership and clear goals and objectives as quintessential to sustaining these movements and point to limitations in these vital areas as reasons for failure. They devote substantial attention to the structuring of protest and the critical role of leaders in that process. Each of the four movements they discuss, the unemployed workers' movement, the industrial workers movement, the Civil Rights Movement, and the welfare rights movement shared positive objectives and mission. However, they failed to grasp the opportunity for real change because of their leaders' doctrinal commitment to the development of mass-based, permanent organization building that forced the masses away from streets and into the meeting rooms (Piven & Cloward, 1979).

If we are to assume the definition of a social movement as "a formally organized group that acts consciously with some continuity to provide or resist change through collective action" (Goldberg, 1991, pp. 1-2), then such a body would require a coherent internal structure, leadership, a written statement of purpose, membership, successful resource mobilization, and a logistical base. Moreover, movements have an ideology that offers their members and leaders a blueprint for promoting or resisting change. Certainly, the million marches have some of these characteristics such as a leadership, the ability to attract large numbers of followers to its marches, and a set of objectives in order to respond to such issues as deficiencies in the American political economy and the problem of White supremacy. However, despite the capacity of the leadership to bring millions of people together on Washington, D.C. and elsewhere, objective factors and the level of disquiet appear insufficient to transform it into a mass movement on the local level.

The matter of leadership is crucial to understanding and defining a social movement. Leadership for the million marches is essentially Black nationalist. Albeit these nationalists for the most part, particularly in 2005, reached out and embraced the integrationist leadership class, the present quest for movement is different from what occurred in the Civil Rights Movement. Nationalists did not play a role in the Civil Rights Movement until the emergence of Black power which made its appearance after much of the civil rights gains had been legislated by the United States Congress.

The Civil Rights Movement of the fifties and sixties achieved intellectual and organizational clarity in what it sought to accomplish.

Differences existed between the Southern Christian Leadership Conference, the National Association of Colored People, the Student Non-Violent Coordinating Committee, and the Congress of Racial Equality. The unity of purpose centered around the destruction of the Jim Crow system and the fact that the most efficacious strategy was mass mobilization of the community and using non-violence to disrupt the Jim Crow equilibrium.

Martin Luther King, Jr. used non-violence and the moral creed of the movement to discredit the oppressive Jim Crow system. There was no reluctance on the part of the Jim Crow officials to use the necessary force to put down the resistance. What made the non-violent tactic so effective was the federal government's willingness to act and to neutralize the excesses of the Jim Crow state apparatus. It was mass mobilization that forced Congress to pass the 1964 Civil Rights Bill and the 1965 Voting Rights Act. Both legislations were instrumental in collapsing the official pillars of Jim Crow governments. The accomplishments of the Civil Rights Movement were historic but modest in changing the material well-being of the Black community.

Martin Luther King, Jr. recognized the achievements of the Civil Rights Movement and understood that in order to build on that success, it was necessary to change the marginalization of the Black community. In the same way that the political system accommodated the demands of the Civil Rights Movement, King, in embarking on the Poor People's Campaign, wanted the poor to be accommodated within the capitalist economic system. King would eventually find out that the struggle for economic inclusion would meet with greater resistance than the struggle to desegregate the South. Martin Luther King, Jr. was assassinated in 1968, the same year that Kevin Phillips identified the emerging Republican majority. The political shift with the election of Richard Nixon, Jimmy Carter, and Ronald Reagan put an end to the struggle for economic inclusion. The number of Black elected officials had increased on the state and on the federal level, but there was no Black mass movement and the justice agenda was placed on the back burner of American politics.

Just as Martin Luther King, Jr. personified the Civil Rights Movement, Louis Farrakhan has epitomized the million march events. The Civil Rights Movement did not begin in Washington with a march. It built around the indignities of Jim Crow that Black people faced on a day to day basis. The Civil Rights Movement which evolved from the ground and mass mobilization took place in different parts of the South. The March on Washington was the culmination of local struggles.

Although the million march events were built around local organiz-ing committees, the reason for their existence was to mobilize people for the marches in Washington. D.C. After the march, the local organiz-ing committees atrophied as there were no local issues to sustain their existence despite the panoply of issues outlined in the 1995 and 2005 march documents.

Farrakhan has the prestige in the Black community to assemble mil-lions, but he lacks the organizational ability to build a mass political movement. He is a religious leader with an apocalyptic vision to solving issues and his religious base has traditionally looked askance at political engagement. It is not surprising that nothing transformative has emerged from the intermittent assembly of millions. The Million/More Movement remains stillborn.

CONCLUSION

The Black community does not take its queues from mainstream me-dia. The distinctive nature of the Black historical experience gives the Black community some autonomy from what passes as American con-ventional wisdom. There has emerged in the Black community a sensi-tivity to the vicissitudes of racism, and the tradition of mass protest is embedded in the political arsenal of the community. From World War II when A. Phillip Randolph threatened to march on Washington, D.C. if President Roosevelt did not take action against job discrimination in the munition industry, the March on Washington has become an essential weapon for the Black community.

President Roosevelt was forced by Randolph to issue an executive order banning discrimination in federal employment, and Randolph called off the March. The March on Washington in 1963 demonstrated the seriousness of the Black community to achieve first class citizen-ship, and that march and organizing mobilization brought about the *de jure* demise of Jim Crow.

The anxiety in the Black community triggered by the right hand drift in American politics prompted Louis Farrakahan to resurrect the mass protest of the March on Washington. Despite the hostility in the mass media to Farrakhan, Black men in the tens of thousands descended on Washington, D.C. in October, 1995. They knew that something had gone amiss in American society. The Black inner city was damaged by the deindustrialization, and America's response to the surplus labor prob-lem was to expand exponentially the incarcerated population inasmuch as Black folk constitute a disproportionate percentage of those who are incarcerated. The Million Man March led by Farrakhan was a statement to the nation that change from within and without was desperately needed.

The Million Women March in 1997 in Philadelphia was an opportunity for females to protest their condition in America. There was the need to strengthen the Black family and to improve the employment possibilities of Black women in the workplace. The Million Youth March that followed in Atlanta and New York failed to capture the imagination of the youth population.

When Louis Farrakhan called for the 2005 Million More March, the leader of the Nation of Islam recognized the need to be inclusive and was cognizant as to how much America in terms of race relations and in relationship to the world had changed. The 2005 organizing document mentioned the need to bring together the multi-racial and multi-cultural base that constituted twenty-first century America.

The Marches on Washington and elsewhere from 1995-2005 have failed to create a social movement in the national Black community. The Marches were not an organized outgrowth of grassroots protest, and after the mass assembling of people, the marches became an end to mobilization rather than the beginning for further political struggle. That was not the case with the Civil Rights Movement. The 1963 March On Washington was an outgrowth of civil rights struggles taking place throughout the South. The March in 1963 was put together specifically to draw the attention of the President and Congressional leaders to pass legislation that would put an end to the nefarious Jim Crow system. Those objectives were accomplished with the passage of the 1964 Civil Rights legislation and the 1965 Voters Rights Act. On the other hand, the objectives of the millions marches on Washington and elsewhere between 1995 and 2005 lacked a clear legislative objective.

Over that ten year span, the millions marches leadership has failed to have an impact on the larger American society. Black folk are troubled by the development of an illiberal punitive form of capitalism that is becoming increasingly coercive in domestic and foreign policy. The preoccupation with praetorianism is a response to the decline in American hegemony in the world. In the post-2005 Million More March period, America has become preoccupied with the whereabouts of 12 million undocumented aliens, and the omnipresence of the terrorist threat. Black people sense the new uneasiness in America and nonetheless, there has failed to emerge a Black grassroots protest movement.

REFERENCES

Campbell, H. (1997). The million women march. (a brief piece prepared for the *SAPEM* a Zimbabwean publication and *Agenda* a South African publication).

Cha-Jua, S. K. & Lang, C. (1997). Providence, patriarchy, pathology: The rise & decline of Louis Farrakhan. *New Politics*, 6 (2) (Winter 1997), 47-71.

Cottman, M. H. (1995). *Million man march*. New York: Crown Trade Paperbacks.

Gladwell, M. (1988). Just say wait a minute. Review essay on, *The Fix*, by Michael Massing, *Drug Crazy: How We Got into the mess and how we can get out,* by Mike Gray. *The New York Review of Books*. (Dec. 17), pp. 4-8.

Goldberg, R. A. (1991). *Grassroots resistance: Social movements in twentieth century America*. Belmont, CA.: Wasdworth.

Green, C. & Wilson, B. (1992). *The struggle for Black empowerment in New York City: Beyond the politics of pigmentation*. New York: Praeger/Greenwood Press (1989); McGraw-Hill (paperback, 1992).

Interview with Dr. Blakely on the million women march in Harlem, N.Y., February, 1999.

Interview with Minister Conrad Muhammad on the youth march and the new hip-hop movement in Harlem, N.Y., February, 1999.

Karenga, M. (1995). The Million Man March/Day of Absence Mission Statement. *The Black Scholar*, 25 (4) (Fall). pp. 2-11.

Kornblum, W. (1997). *Sociology in a changing world*. 4th Edition. New York: Harcourt, Brace.

Kornhauser, W. (1959). *The politics of mass society*. New York: Free Press.

LeBon, G. (1947/1896). *The crowd*. London: Ernest Bonn.

Lipset, S. (1959). *Political man: The social bases of politics*. Garden city, NY: Doubleday.

Luneskas, J. (1998). "Another Successful AR Conference", Internet).

Massing, M. (Nov. 19, 1988). The Blue Revolution, a review essay of three books: *How America's top cop reversed the crime epidemic* by: William Bratton; *Getting away with murder: how politics is destroying the criminal justice system;* by: Susan Estrich; *Politics, Punishment and Population* by: Lord Winglesham. *The New York Review of Books,* 45 (18), pp. 32-36.

McCormick, J. (1997). The messages and the messengers: Opinions from the million men who marched. *The National Political Science Review*, (6), 142-164.

Moss, M., Townsend, A., & Tobien, E. (1997). *Immigration is Transforming New York City*. The Taub Urban Research Center, New York University.

Noel, P. (1998). Minister of War. *New York*. (September 7), pp. 22-27.

Phillips, K. (1969). *The Emerging Republican Majority*. New York: Arlington House.

Piven, F. F. & Cloward, R. (1979). *Poor People's Movements: Why The Succeed, How They Fail*. New York: Vintage.

Robinson, C. (1997). *Black movements in America*. New York: Routledge.

Sadler, K. M. (Ed). (1996). *Atonement: The Million Man March*. Cleveland, OH: The Pilgrim Press.

Smelser, N. (1962). *Theory of Collective Behavior*. New York: Free Press.

Schooling and Globalization: What Do We Tell Our Kids & Clients? What Are We Being Told?

Carl A. Grant

Alicia Grant

INTRODUCTION

Rapid advances in information technology have turned the world into a global village, making globalization, which was previously an economic ideology, a multi-faceted fact of life that increasingly affects what we do, including what we eat, what kinds of jobs we hold, and how much we know about what's happening outside the borders of our own nation. It is also affecting education and schools. So what do we as educators and social workers tell our kids (as well as our clients, the parents of the kids we serve) about the effects of globalization?

These two questions frame our discussion in this article about schooling and globalization. Implicit in both questions is a concern about social justice, a political philosophy that serves as our theoretical lens. To begin, we will first define globalization and social justice. This is followed by (1) a rationale for examining globalization; (2) a discussion of the methodology and procedures we used for the informal study we conducted in conjunction with this paper; (3) a discussion about what we learned from this study; and (4) some recommendations about what we should tell out kids about globalization.

DEFINITIONS

Globalization

The definitions of globalization we use come from Jill Blackmore (2000) who sees globalization as ". . . increased economic, cultural, environmental, and social interdependencies and new transnational financial and political formation arising out of the mobility of capital, labor and information, with both homogenizing and differentiating tendencies" (p. 33). Blackmore's definition is consistent with what the International Monetary Fund (IMF) considers the four aspects of globalization: trade, capital movement, movement of people, and the spread of knowledge (and technology). Malcolm Waters (1995) provides another definition of globalization that is significant to our response and our use of social justice as a theoretical lens, because it takes into account the influence of Western societies on globalization. Waters argues that, "Globalization is the direct consequence of the expansion of European culture across the planet via settlement, colonization and cultural mimesis. It is also bound up intrinsically with the pattern of capitalist development as it has ramified through political and cultural arenas" (p. 2). However,

Walters also notes that, "This does not imply that every corner of the planet must become Westernized and capitalist but rather that every set of social arrangements must establish its position in relation to the capitalist West." (p. 3).

Social Justice

For this article, we consider social justice as "fairness" (Rawls, 1957), which takes into account the treatment of inequalities of all kinds (e.g., the elimination of institutionalized domination and oppression); and, as such, embraces equity in the distribution of a wide range of attributes. Here we are not only referring to material things, but less tangible things such as equal opportunity and access. In addition, social justice contends individuals should not be advantaged or disadvantaged by natural fortune or social circumstance (e.g., race, gender, socio economic status) in choice of principles (Barry, 2005).

In many countries, increasing globalization has meant that schooling/education is associated with two areas where social justice is of paramount significance: one, distributive justice or material equality, and two, cultural justice. In developing countries, distributive justice might mean something as fundamental as having a school building and the opportunity to attend school regularly. In the United States, distributive justice would, for instance, mean students who live in urban and rural areas have schools that are equal (e.g., qualified teachers and resources) to schools in the suburban areas (Kozol, 1991, 1995). Cultural justice necessitates treating all people as equal, regardless of characteristics such as race, color, nationality, or language.

RATIONALE: PUTTING A FACE ON THE PROBLEM

As an educator and an aspiring social worker, we are concerned with this topic, because discourse about globalization and its effects are all around us. Here we are referring to discussions in the media, as well as discussions we have with our friends and family members, about the effects of globalization. These effects include the boom in the technology field; the draining of the best and brightest minds from other countries; outsourcing; the movement in education from a bureaucratic to a market form of governance; rising gas prices; international political instability and upheavals such as the revival of ethnic- and religious-based nationalist movements; and an observation that internationally education is becoming more convergent.

In addition, we became concerned with this topic because of what we saw was available in print media about the effects of globalization when we visited a consumer magazine and periodical section at a local book store to assess how the general public is being informed about schooling and globalization. This visit was inspired because we noticed that globalization is only receiving narrow attention in the school curriculum (Gough, 1999).

Perhaps the fundamental reason behind our concerns are Alicia's children (and my grandchildren) Gavin, 10, and Amaya, 4. We all live together in an upper middle class community with good schools. Living the lifestyle we do—American middle-class—many of the prequisites of the effects globalization (e.g., multiple technologies, cheaper prices on goods due to outsourcing and international trade) are available to us. The headaches of the effects globalization (e.g., global warming, rivalry among states for control of natural resources, the ignoring of developing countries that have little to contribute to globalization) come our way too, but their immediate effects on us are somewhat mediated by the government and our socio-economic position.

What we're getting at is that it's not Gavin and Amaya that we have the great worries about (although perhaps we should, and we each do have some worries), but that as a family we are worried about the children who live in underdeveloped or less industrialized countries throughout the world, as well as the poor urban and rural areas in the United States. These children are vulnerable to a global economy and culture rooted in North American and Western interests and ideas. Also, the public school—that is, receiving an education, and here we are speaking about a college education—which was at one time considered the instrument of social mobility, is increasingly becoming less accessible as public education becomes increasingly privatized, and this privitization reform exacerbates inequalities related to social class and race (Lipman, 2004; Smith, 2004).

METHODOLOGY AND PROCEDURE

Being haunted by the questions: "What do we tell our kids about globalization?" and "What are members of the general public–including we as parents, teachers, and social workers–being told about globalization and how it affects schooling and education?" we decided on a plan of action to attempt to answer those questions. At the time this was personal, not professional. Then, a journal editor presented us with the opportunity to make this story professional. Thus, our methods and procedures are not those prescribed in research methods texts. Nevertheless, we suggest that you not dismiss what we discovered.

Method

Our method was based upon discovering what consumers at a large, international chain of book stores would find in the periodical and magazine section about globalization and schooling. The book store we chose was Borders. From our observations, Borders stocks and displays a wide variety of consumer magazine and periodicals. In addition, the Borders we used is located in a city that is home to the state capital and a world class university.

On April 25, 2006 and May 29, 2007, we visited the Borders book store in our community and examined the magazine and periodical section. In April of 2006 we found three articles where "global" (or some synonym) was in the title of the article. We are not saying that some of the other articles did not have references to globalization, but a review showed they were not directly related to our purpose. The three articles we found are:

- "Curbing Global Corruption" by Ben W. Heineman, Jr. and Fritz Heineman, *Foreign Affairs* (May/June 2006)
- "The Globally Integrated Enterprise" by Samuel J. Palmisano, *Foreign Affairs* (May/June 2006)
- "Global Delusions," (a review of three books: *Globalization and Its Enemies* by Daniel Cohen; *How We Compete: What Companies Around the World Are Doing to Make It in Today's Global Economy*, by Suzanne Berger; and *End of the Line: The Rise and Coming Fall of the Global Corporation* by Barry C. Lynn) by John Gray, *New York Review of Books* (April 27, 2006).

In May 29, 2007 we found six articles:

- "Beyond American Hegemony" by Michael Lind, *The National Interest* (May/June 2007)
- "Losing Mythic Authority" by Michael Vlabos, *The National Interest* (May/June 2007)

- "A Goldilocks World Economy?" by Sherle R. Schwenninger, *World Policy Journal* (Winter, 2006/2007)
- "Prison Planet" by Roy Walmsley, *Foreign Policy* (May/June 2007)
- "Raising the Stakes" by Joshua Kurlantzick, *Foreign Policy* (May/June 2007)
- "Inside the Digital Dump" by Natalie Behring, *Foreign Policy* (May/June 2007)

Procedure and Analysis

After discovering the nine articles, we reviewed them to discover if and how schooling/education and globalization were discussed (e.g., connection, intersection, level of complexities). Because of space limitations, we will only discuss four of them in detail in this paper.

The Heineman and Heineman article "Curbing Global Corruption" reports on global corruption and argues that, although nations have enacted anticorruption laws, and international business groups have promulgated model codes of behavior, the "international media reports instances of corruption in high places virtually everyday" (p. 75). The article concludes with the argument that an anticorruption movement needs to be started, one that contends, "Ultimately, the most potent force for change is the idea that corruption is morally repugnant and inimical to competition, globalization, the rule of law, international development, and the welfare of citizens around the world" (p. 86).

Samuel F. Palmisano, Chair of the Board, President, and Chief Executive Officer of IBM, in "The Globally Integrated Enterprise" proclaims that there is a new kid on the block in globalization–"the globally integrated enterprise." He invites the reader to be supportive of this idea. Palmisano states, "[B]usinesses are changing in fundamental ways–structurally, operationally, culturally–in response to the imperatives of globalization and new technology" (p. 127). Palmisano goes on to argue that "rather than continuing to focus on past models, regulators, scholars, nongovernmental organizations, community leaders and business executives would be best served by thinking about global corporations of the future and its implication for new approaches to regulation, education, trade and commerce" (p. 127-128). Palmisano addresses education in the article as follows:

> The single most important challenge in shifting to globally integrated enterprises–and the consideration driving most business decision

today–will be securing a supply of high-value skills. Nations and companies alike must invest in better basic educational and training programs (p. 133-134).

At the conclusion of his article Palmisano states:

The globally integrated enterprise is a promising new actor on the world stage. Now leaders in business, government, education, and all of civil society must learn about its emerging dynamics and help it mature in ways that will contribute to social, and economic, and human progress round the planet (p. 136).

John Gray's review of the three books: *Globalization and Its Enemies*; *How We Compete: What Companies Around the World Are Doing to Make It in Today's Global Economy*; and *End of the Line: The Rise and Coming Fall of the Global Corporation* is a thorough critique, which for the most part individually, but especially collectively, considers IMF's four aspects of globalization: trade, capital movement, movement of people, and the spread of knowledge (and technology). On reading Gray's review you come away with a richer insight into globalization. It includes a historical overview of globalization that dates backs to the sixteenth century with the conquistadors' arrival in the New World and continued in the nineteenth century with British imperial free trade. We learned that: (1) the nineteen-century globalization involved large-scale movements of people to new lands, while the present phase involves mainly commodities and images; (2) the reason poor countries stay poor is that they have little that rich countries want or need and the poor of the world are not so much exploited as neglected and forgotten; and (3) the fundamental forces driving globalization are a great free up of trade and capital flows; deregulation; the shrinking cost of communication and transportation; an information technology revolution that makes it possible to digitize data and blur the boundaries between design, manufacturing and marketing, thus enabling corporations to locate these functions in different places; and the availability of large numbers of workers and engineers in low-wage countries.

Sherle R. Schwenninger's "A Goldilocks World Economy?" argues that the United States should work toward an economy that is "not to hot, not too cold, but just right." Schwenninger contends that with the integration of China, India, and the former Soviet Union into the global economy, along with the technology advancement and other changes which have substantially increased U.S. and world productivity growth, a new abundance has been created. This new abundance, Schwenniger claims, has created the conditions for more rapid economic growth and rising living standards. However in order to take advantages of these condition, Schwenniger argues the U. S. must put in place a "public investment strategy." According to Schwenniger the strategy:

> [R]ather than encouraging emerging economies to develop primarily though the export of manufactured goods and their compo-nents parts, U. S. international economic policy should champion middle-class development aimed at increasing domestic consump-tion. This means help emerging economies to expand home own-ership invest in public infrastructure, **improve public education**, build a social safety net, and create more small and medium-size business–much as the Untied States did in the last century (p. 7; emphasis added).

DISCUSSION

The articles we read on the effects of globalization address trade, cap-ital movement, movement of people, the spread of technology, and the inclusion of China, India and the former Soviet Union as principal actors with only a narrow discussion of schooling/education. When schooling/ education is discussed in relation to globalization, it is not defined and/or the discussion tends to focus on the necessity and preparation of a skilled work force in our technological society. Azad's (2004) obser-vation is illustrative of what one often finds, "An important component of globalization in relation to [*sic*] education is the need for producing higher quality manpower that can successfully face competition in the world markets. This would imply selecting the best possible human ma-terial and giving them education of highest quality" (p. 9).

Implicit in most discussions of globalization and education is the be-lief that schooling/education is doing a poor job of preparing workers for a globalized society. In other words, members of the American pub-lic selecting a periodical or magazine from Borders during that the two months used in our examples will probably come away with a very poor perception of how schools are preparing students for the effects of glob-alization and a narrow understanding of the role of schooling/education in our global society. Enhancing this perception is an understanding that over the past two and half decades, starting with the report *A Nation at Risk: The Imperative for Educational Reform,* released in 1983 by the

National Commission on Excellence in Education, government officials and business leaders have been highly critical of public education. *A Nation at Risk* states:

> If an unfriendly foreign power had attempted to impose on America the mediocre educational performance that exists today, we might well have viewed it as an act of war. As it stands, we have allowed this to happen to ourselves. We have even squandered the gain in student achievement made in the wake of the Sputnik challenge. Moreover, we have dismantled essential support systems which help to make those gains possible. We have in effect, committed an act of unthinking unilateral educational disarmament (p. 5).

More recently, Neubauer (2005) argued that classroom life remains pretty much the same as it did decades ago. Instruction is highly structured; ability grouping and segregation by age remains firmly in place; and textbooks hold sway over what is taught and how it is taught. In other words, "One could argue that we are continuing to organize education to train and educate people to work and succeed in a world that increasingly no longer exists" (Neubauer, 2005, p. 3).

Such an observation in this period of increased globalization no doubt leaves the ordinary person, including parents of kids in school, angry with public education and anxious and confused about what to tell their children about schooling/education and globalization. In addition, and central to the point of this article, is that such observations leave them with only half of the story. True, public schools in the United States need a great deal of serious work As we mention above, one only has to read Jonathan Kozol's two books, written with the American public in mind to learn that schooling/education needs a great deal of work. *Savage Inequalities: Children in America's Schools* (1991) and *The Shame of the Nation: The Restoration of Apartheid Schooling in America* (2005) by Kozol make it crystal clear that schooling/education in the United States, especially in urban areas, is shameful (e.g., old buildings, need for more highly qualified teachers, more technology).

The other half of the story that we are addressing in our observations about schooling/education and the effects globalization is the absence of discussions about of what some call a "new humanism" or social justice. The Delors Commission (1996) states

> Education should help engender a new humanism that contains an essential ethical component and set considerable store by

knowledge of, and respect for the culture and spiritual values of different civilizations, as much needed counter weight to globalization that
would otherwise be seen only in economical or technological terms (p.
2).

In addition to a new humanism, which we believe is essential, there is
need for an analytical discussion of schooling/education and the effects
of globalization within a civic context. By civic context, we are referring to Thomas Jefferson's notion that we need an informed citizenry to
make the democratic government work –and, we hasten to add, we need
informed citizens in this age of globalization, perhaps now more than
ever. The reasons are:

• Since globalization is redefining and/or influencing the role of the
  nation state as a manager, as well as how it manages political, economic and relations between and among nation states, attention
  needs to be given to democratic principles and procedures at the
  local, state, and community level, including involving (more) people in the democratic process beyond just voting every two to four
  years. If not, it will limit citizens' abilities to develop understanding and knowledge and have voice which they can use to mediate
  the strong, objectionable effects of globalization. This way of
  thinking assigns schooling/education a significant role in the creation of active and informed citizens who resist being treated
  (only) as either objects of globalized economic activity or as consumers of globalized cultural symbols and products. Education in
  both developed and developing countries is increasingly directed
  toward economic and vocational goals with the aim of producing
  workers who have the skills and disposition to assist countries in
  successfully competing in the global economy. Nelly Stromquist
  and Karen Monkman (2000) have observed: ". . . education is losing
  ground as a public good to become rather a marketable commodity.
  The state has become limited in its responsibility to schooling, often guaranteeing basic education, but extracting in turn user fees
  from higher levels of public education, as any other service in the
  market . . . The new outlook has made social policy secondary to the
  market and has 'atomized the social,' centering on the interests of
  the individual as consumer rather than as citizen" (pp. 12-13, 15).
  In addition, education is becoming commoditized and transformed
  into a service. Such developments are changing the focus of
  educational knowledge and practices away from social and cultural

concerns (for example, the arts in schools are increasingly neglected) to those of individuals and economies in which they participate. Paradoxically, the emphasis on skills for employment comes at a time when many post-secondary students are facing difficulty finding decent jobs. Many of the jobs available mainly pay cost-of-living wages, and many of them permit workers to work only half-time in order for the employer to avoid paying health insurance. In addition, many post secondary students have difficulty attending college because of high tuition rates, the lack of college loans, and the increased selectivity of applicants based upon grade-point-average.

- With globalization, come new economic and social problems and issues such as wage migration (e.g., guest workers), conflict over ideas regarding gender equity, and ethnic and religious polarization within and across some countries. Nation states can more successfully address problems of cultural difference and financial inequalities with a citizenry that has learned how to analyze and critique problems or issues.
- Educational systems, besides becoming the whipping child for globalization, have become the sites of cultural wars. A growing number of ethnographic studies report that schools are increasingly becoming sites of cultural battles over language, religion, dress, ethnicity, social class, race, and attitude and behavior in the classroom (e.g., model minority versus hip and cool). Contestation– between national chauvinism, traditional representations of the nation-state, and increased signs and symbols from citizens representing different abilities and lifestyles who are demanding to exercise the full capacity of citizenship–is being increased.
- Finally, schooling/education which has been (and is) vital to the creation of the students' identity and self concept, as well as influencing perceptions of others about individuals and groups of people, will be need to play an active role in positive identity formation in order to help students successfully handle the effects of globalization.

WHAT WE SHOULD TELL OUR KIDS

We should tell our kids to use their schooling to learn the 3Rs, and to learn tools of analysis which will help them to investigate/interrogate the problems and issues that will be ever-changing during their lifetimes because of the effects of globalization upon society, themselves, and others who live on the margin. We must help them to become aware that the educational system is increasingly being forced into a market mode and that there is movement away from the traditional–although yet unachieved–notion of education in the public interest, for the general welfare and social good, with attention on the "whole" individual.

Simply put, we must tell our kids they must acquire an education that will help them to become active and informed citizens who resist being treated as either objects of globalized economic activity or as consumers of globalized cultural products.

REFERENCES

Azad, J. L. (2004). Globalization and Its Impact on Education, [electronic version] cie.du.ac.in/Globalization%20and%20Its%20Impact%20on%20Education%20Basu%20Memorial%20lecture%202004.doc

Barry, B. (2005). Why social justice matters. Cambridge: Polity Press.

Blackmore, J. (1999). Localization/globalization and the midwife state: Strategic dilemmas for state feminism in education. *Journal of Education Policy*, Vol, 14, 1, 33-54.

Card, D. & Krueger, A. B. (1992). Does school quality matter? Returns to education and the characteristics of public schools in the United States. *Journal of Political Economy*. University of Chicago Press, vol. 100(1), pages, 1-40 February.

Delors, Jacques et al. (1996). Learning, The Treasure Within: Report to UNESCO of the International Commission on Education for the Twenty-first Century. Paris: UNESCO.

Gough, Noel. (1999). Globalization and school curriculum change: Locating a transnational imaginary. *Journal Educational Policy*, 14, 1, 73-84.

Gray, J. (2006). *The New York Review of Books,* "Global Delusions" *Globalization and Its Enemies* by Daniel Cohen; *How we Compete: What Companies Around the World Are doing to Make It in Today's Global Economy, by* Suzanne Berger; and *End of the Line: The Rise and Coming Fall of the Global Corporation* by Barry C. Lynn.

Heineman, B. W. Jr. & Heineman, F. (May/June 2006)."Curbing Global Corruption." *Foreign Affairs*.

Henry, M., Lingard, B. Rizvi, F., & Taylor, S. (1999). Working with/against globalization in education. *Journal of Education Policy*, Vol, 14, 185,185-197.

Kozol, J. (1991). *Savage Inequalities: Children in America's Schools*. New York: Harper Collins.

Limman, P. (2004). High stakes education: Inequality, globalization and urban school reform. New York: Routledge.

National Commission on Excellence in Education, *A Nation at Risk: The Imperative for Educational Reform.* Washington D. C.: Author, 1983.

Neubauer, D. (2005). Globalization, interdependence and education. Paper presented to the International Seminar on "Education in China: The Dialectics of the Global and the Local," November 15, 2005.

Palmisano, S. J. (May/June, 2006). "The Globally Integrated Enterprise." *Foreign Affairs*.

Rawls, J. (1957). Justice as fairness. *Journal of Philosophy*, 54, October, 653-662.

Smith, D. M. (1994). Geography and social justice. Cambridge, MA: Blackwell.

Smith, M. L. (2004). Political spectacle and the fate of American schools. New York: Routledge.

Stromquist, N. P. & Mondman, K. (Editors). (2000). Globalization and education: Integration and contestation across cultures. 2nd Edition. Lanham, MD: Rowman & Littlefield.

Waters, Malcolm. (1995). Globalization and its discontents: New York: Routledge.

Young, I. M. (1990). Justice and the politics of differences. Princeton, N.J.: Princeton University Press.

REFLECTIONS ON THE EVOLUTION OF RACE CONSCIOUSNESS ACROSS THREE GENERATIONS OF SOCIAL WORK EDUCATORS

A Journey Through the Prism of Race:
An Evolution of Generational Consciousness

June G. Hopps
Elaine Pinderhughes
Tony B. Lowe

INTRODUCTION

Three colleagues, eighty, sixty, and forty something, look back over their personal growth and development as professionals. Their experiences, through years apart, are more similar than dissimilar, demonstrating that systems change is hard, but critical, if all Americans are to have an opportunity for real economic advancement and self-actualization. By following their personal experiences, the prism of race (or race consciousness) is one way that many might learn how to interpret their daily lives. Through the reflective observations of these professors, over four score years of personal, historical and professional change is noted, albeit briefly.

One author is a former Dean and Professor of the School of Social Work (SSW) at Boston College, Editor-in-Chief of *Social Work*, past Chair of the Board of Trustees and a Life Trustee at Spelman College, and currently the Parham Professor at the University of Georgia (UGA). Another is a professor who has made great contributions to the literature in the clinical domain, chaired the clinical sequence at Boston College SSW for years, and was appointed as the Moses Professor at Hunter College, Rappaport Professor at Smith College, and the Lucille Austin Professor at Columbia University, and finally, one is an assistant professor at the UGA in the SSW and is developing a record of scholarship on race, social work practice, mental health policy, and workplace violence.

EARLY MESSAGES:
FAMILIES, SCHOOLS, AND COMMUNITIES

Elaine's Perspective

The shape of diversity consciousness in my life was determined by the fact that I had grown up in a warm, comfortable, sheltered, middle class, and very stable community in Washington, D.C., with excellent though segregated schools. Thus, the enigma and injustice associated with being African American was for the most part distant although never completely absent. My father was a dentist, and our parents' friends and neighbors were primarily professionals and government workers. In school we were taught many facts about our history that could not be found in our textbooks, particularly about the many unacknowledged achievements of Negroes or Colored people as we were identified in those days. Interestingly, the emphasis was not on racism—we did not even use that word—but on presenting models of success and on instilling discipline along with the values of hard work, collaboration, and commitment to "being a credit to the race."

These goals were reinforced by events such as the annual Elks Oratorical Contest in which high school students debated governmental enforcement of the rights granted to Negroes by the 13th, 14th and 15th Amendments to the Constitution. The students' speeches were fiery, passionate and inspiring as they examined the amendments and their failed implementation. But while our parents and teachers tried, they could not shield us from the horrors being committed against the Negro people. I had learned to read on the headlines of the local African American newspapers (the *Washington Afro-American* and the *Pittsburgh Courier*) at a time when there was at least one lynching a week and on the long descriptions of the repeated failures of Congress to pass an anti-lynching bill, because the Southern block always succeeded in filibustering it to death.

Upon reflection, it was against the background of stability, safety, and support so solidly supplied by our families, friends, teachers, churches, and community that I began to question from my earliest days the contradictions and inconsistencies that plagued the meaning I was seeking to construct about diversity, about what it meant to be Colored, Negro, Afro-American, African-American, Black.

It started in my family as I struggled to understand the skin color prejudice of Negroes that I sensed as a young child. I was sensitized to it early because my father was so dark and my mother so fair, being frequently mistaken for White even by other Negroes, and always, or so it seemed to me, considered as movie-star beautiful. I was confused that it was forbidden in our house to refer to anyone in terms of skin color (such as that light-skinned girl or that dark skinned boy). To me this was merely commenting on an obvious fact; however I later came to see it was my parents' (ill-conceived) attempt to cope with the poison of skin color prejudice.

However, my mother's fair skin saved my father from economic ruin when, during the Depression, he had so few patients that the family was in serious financial jeopardy, and my mother passed to secure a job (and economic security) she could never have held had it been known that she was Negro. While at the time I deeply resented her rescue efforts as pushing her into a world I could not enter, I have later reflected on the extraordinary courage this required from both of them, especially my father, given his sense of pride.

I also recall my confusion that our music teacher would teach her Black pupils to sing the song, "Rule Britannia, Britannia rule the waves, Britons never, never, never will be slaves!" And we, little Negro children, sang these poisonous lyrics with gusto, never considering the vulnerability to self denigration that they implied.

Indelibly etched in my memory is the day that the White neighborhood pharmacist who often filled prescriptions of my fathers' patients, growled as we sought to order ice cream sodas, "Take your black paws off the counter!" I remember the sense of pride I felt when our father immediately took us back to witness his furious response to this insult to his daughters, including his vow to send his patients elsewhere. We spread the word in the neighborhood and never again entered that establishment.

June's Perspective

I grew up in Central Florida (Ocala, Marion County) on Gary Farms, a cattle farm owned initially by my paternal grandparents, William P. Gary and Mamie Elizabeth Harvey Gary. My parents, Ollie Colden Gary and Homer Gary, raised me and my four siblings on one parcel of the farm that extended a mile in each direction. The "mile" is important in our lives, because bonding among the five of us took place on long walks or pony rides, especially to the pond, grape arbor, and plum trees. Both of our parents were active in the community, which during that era was segregated, including most farm/business dealings.

My grandfather, Pa'pa, was a beloved, instrumental figure in the lives of his five grandchildren; four girls in a row and one boy, the youngest child. Before he became ill and infirm, he had taught me and two of my sisters how to read, ride a pony, count, add and subtract, how to sit still and listen in Sunday school, church, and funerals where final respect was paid to family members, friends, and neighbors, who were usually laid out in some shade of purple. We were taught the value of property ownership and assets early on and never ever to sell the family holdings. We all learned well. My maternal grandmother, Lucy Shannon Colden (wife of Lee Colden, my maternal grandfather), visited often and spent her time teaching us our prayers and the meaning of religious faith. Spiritual and outgoing, she helped out in home chores of canning and preserving fruits and vegetables. She rocked whomever was the baby, all the time.

Learning to read under Pa'pa's tutelage and on his lap in late afternoon, except during the winter months, was a favorite and engaging time for exploring the wonders of a world beyond the pastures, rural district roads, and a small town. We learned about Washington, D.C., the capital city, New York City, the Japanese who bombed Pearl Harbor, Adolph Hitler, Joseph Stalin, Joe Louis, Jackie Robinson, but especially civil and human rights topics covered by both the White and Colored print media during that period with special attention to the differential emphasis on the same subjects. Additionally, there were books in our mother's small, but important collection. That selection included works by or about Paul Lawrence Dunbar, Phyllis Wheatley, W.E.B. Du Bois, Booker T. Washington, Mary McLeod Bethune, George Washington Carver, Richard Allen, the Roosevelt's, Shakespeare, Tennyson, Browning, Abraham Lincoln, and Benjamin Mays, who wrote a column in the *Pittsburgh Courier* (a national Black newspaper), to cite only a few. The main books were Bibles, of course. My grandfather would read them. He would also read our Sunday School lessons and review them with us as well as our early text books. In essence, he guaranteed his grandchildren a *head start:* Four granddaughters earned doctorates at early ages and his only grandson is the manager of Gary Farms.

Starting school was not very eventful; I could read a little, count and write my name thanks to Pa'pa for his wisdom, guidance, and loving patience. Further, since my mother was a teacher at Howard Academy, I was not really getting away from her influence and instruction nor going to a new, challenging environment since I had been in and out of her classroom on many occasions for most of my previous four years of life. In addition, two aunts, one paternal and one maternal, who lived and worked in Marion County, also taught school in small communities, or hamlets as we called them, and I spent many days "helping" one aunt teach by doing the "most" important tasks including putting out chalk, erasers, old frayed books that were passed down from the White children, paper, and then collecting all the items, sorting them out and storing them at the end of the school day. The ride home was one where I watched for state patrol cars, polecats, because of their black and cream skunk like color and more significantly, their strong reputation for stopping and mistreating Colored drivers–the few who owned horseless carriages (i.e., automobile or trucks).

Hearing Pa'pa read about events relative to survival of Colored people was not only interesting, but also confusing, contradictory and at times frightening. Discussions about beatings, lynchings, and car bombings of "Coloreds" though whispered among adults when we were very young, was undoubtly the nadir. The secretary at Howard Academy lost both of her parents in South Florida in a fatal car bombing. The entire school and the Colored community were in obviously deep shock and grief. But, the mourning was silent, without public discussion or grief counseling that our profession provides in any traumatic experience today. This type of post traumatic stress was not a part of the culture or nomenclature of the African American social experience. The recovery was dealt with on bowed knees in the sacristy of the church and the privacy of homes.

Voting was an emotional and hot subject of discussion: Why didn't more Colored people vote? Economic and physical repercussion? The inability to understand the questions? Problems getting to the polls? What my parents, grandfather, aunts, and a few of their close associates were alluding to was the fear and intimidation their neighbors, friends, some relatives and others in the Black community surely must have experienced. What was at stake was both physical and economic survival. With a very limited middle class, most men were employed as farm workers, mechanics, and common laborers, and women as domestic servants or laundresses. Most Coloreds worked directly for White people and were afraid of a changing social structure where future roles were unknown in the long-term, and in the short-term, the loss of what income they earned, however inadequate that was. Also, on the surface the races appeared to "get along"–most of the time. True feelings were probably masked as described by Franz Fanon. The behavior Blacks demonstrated might be called both a code of silence and at the same time a wall of fear.

Unions were not organized in the South, so neither Blacks nor Whites were afforded any job protection. Sales and clerk jobs were not available, unless in the limited number of Colored owned business. Many of these businesses where largely those in which Whites refused to operate, because of direct service to the Coloreds, such as embalmer-funeral directors, taxi companies, dry cleaners, insurance sales (i.e., burial), and many personal service professions. In my town, Colored people owned dry good (i.e., clothing) and grocery stores and fairly significant pieces of real estate on a main street, Broadway, and other sites.

No matter how successful households were financially, they faced prejudice and discrimination. The contradiction of the ideal, equality, and reality of a dual conscious scenario that W.E.B. DuBois articulated was ever manifested: How to be first rate in your craft, but at the same time always viewed us a second rate American. I lived in a segregated society. School principals, teachers, preachers, office workers, hair dressers, physicians, dentists, skilled laborers (i.e., carpenters, plumbers, electricians), seamstresses, dry cleaners, school bus drivers, and household and farm workers were Colored. (However, my grandfather and father would hire White seasonal workers for the farm.) These *Colored* individuals were competent, successful, proud people who looked forward to a better day when they could become full participants in a democratic society, vote without fear of being insulted or even killed, paid a salary comparable to that of Whites who did the same job (i.e., teachers, public employees & domestics), and enjoy the freedom to purchase property, build assets, and engage in civil protests. In a word, they wanted their rights. My mother's principal was a bright, brainy, politically savvy man who filed for equal salaries for *Colored* teachers. He had to leave the school system. He established a small business co-op and later moved on to become the Chief Executive Officer of a Black insurance company. He and my parents were close friends. My mother stood with him. The next school year she was quietly reassigned to a rural one room facility, quite a distance from our home. It turns out that she loved the new job, and the students and parents loved her. The lesson for her children was to stand up for your beliefs, even if you have to take a bad knock and a bad rap. Both my grandfather and father were perhaps even more committed to equality and sacrificed much because of their beliefs including loss of property and livestock.

By the time, I was in second grade, I got into trouble with my teacher, because I refused to stand and say the Pledge of Allegiance. Marched down to the principal's office by the teacher, I simply explained what I had heard discussed at home. My Pa'pa thought the teacher was "crazy" (she should have been proud of his oldest grandchild, who understood that the country was not just and certainly, there was not "one nation under God"). How else could you explain the draconian slave system and economy, and the existing, pernicious plight of poor Coloreds and Seminole Indians? A few years later, I was in trouble again because of my discussion of the political battle in the Democratic Party over the Civil Rights platform. In fact, my teacher told me to "sit down, be quiet and do not discuss this again."

By this time, I was aware of the fear that many felt in the battle for rights. The struggle and planning was often silent–it was the same way during slavery. I know it is true because Pa'pa told us how slaves planned their escapes–secretly. He knew that first hand, from his parents. The law governing education was *Plessey v. Ferguson*, separate and *equal*. Not so. What this Supreme Court ruling did was to provide validation for discrimination and the disease of inequality. The school system was separate and unequal. The per capita resource allocations proved this. Pa'pa would purchase our schoolbooks, so that we did not have to use those handed down from White to Colored schools and all marked up with graffiti and other typical youthful expression. Of course, by the time a book reached my younger siblings it was truly a hand-me-down, but the meaning, intent, and historical significance did not reek with the onerous whiff of discrimination and moral inferiority.

Earlier laws, customs, and practices made it essentially impossible for Blacks to pursue an authentic education. In fact, education was criminalized. Just as state legislative bodies, courts, and the White society understood that Black literacy was critical to their collective internal development; Blacks understood that literacy was their people's path to a stronger and more fulfilling future. It is no coincidence then that the new "freedmen," the Freedmen's Bureau, Black legislators of the Reconstruction era, and Northern missionaries developed the South's first, universal public education system.

Community leaders, including the Garys, had been exposed to the teaching of great personalities through Historically Black College Universities (HBCU's) and churches, for the most part segregated as they have been since their time as secret slave organizations. In fact, the Garys were in the vanguard of both the talented tenth and the independent/industrial group so strongly debated by W.E.B. Du Bois and Booker T. Washington. My mother, mostly self-educated though a college graduate, could recite poetry (i.e., Shakespeare, Tennyson, Browning, Hughes, Dunbar) read (speak and sing) a little French, and two of our aunts could play the piano. My grandfather and father were successful in their domains: farming, cattle, and mining businesses.

The Washington (pragmatist)–Du Bois (theoretician) discussion, debate and backstage drama took place regularly in the Gary home among family and friends, though it was years before I identified this dialogue for its historical and practical significance. The older folks had a way of staving off and withholding from their offspring for as long as they could the dreaded reality of second-class citizenship, while at the same time preparing them for first-rate citizens, independent thinkers, economic prosperity, community leadership, and future change agents. Clearly, that was and remains the mission of the Gary family commencing with William Primus (Pa' pa) and Mamie Elizabeth (who died before seeing any of her grandchildren).

Tony's Perspective

Hogansville, a city in the west central rolling hills of Georgia, served as my canvas of racial consciousness. Born in the mid 1960's, surrounding many watershed moments of the Civil Rights movement, the community was the kind of place where everybody supposedly knew their neighbors and did not have to lock their house at night. My orientation toward race consciousness began in this environment.

My earliest memory was of the family "moving." Unknown to me, the family was moving from the predominately Black to the town's "White side of the track." As many towns in the deep South, Hogansville has a railroad track that divides the town into eastern and western hemispheres. What was obvious is that vestiges of racial segregation from a by-gone-era continued–the east end was and is mostly White and west end was and is mostly Black. Socio-economic differences were also obvious in the size, value, and quality of homes, as well as differences in city services. The two large public graveyards also preserved this same racial divide, as the White one was well taken care of by the city and the Black one was poorly maintained. Only recently has the public White cemetery integrated; African Americans are beginning to be buried there, but the poorly maintained Black cemetery remains all Black.

In the meantime, we were the only Black family in the middle of this White community from the late 1960s to the late 1970s. Since our contact with neighbors was rare, we only played with each other and have many wonderful childhood memories for this reason. However, I was able to make some special life long White friends from that period in my life. Notwithstanding the efforts of a few citizens to promote de-segregation, the racial caste of this town was highly pronounced.

Growing up in an attenuated, extended Back family that included my grandmother, mother, siblings, and any number of my aunts, uncles, and my cousins made life interesting. The fact was that others could, and did come home; my grandmother and mother always made room for them. That was an unwritten rule. This was true because we lived in the "home house." In this house, family was always welcome, and no one would dare cast judgment on the rationale for one's return. Although Daniel P. Moynihan in *The Negro Family: The Case for National Action* (1965) framed this practice as a deficit, Andrew Billingsley (1968) in his classic book *The Black Family in White America* re-interpreted the fluidity of family boundaries as a strength. For us, the use of family and close friends as an informal (or natural) helping system of survival was the preferred form of support.

Work was clearly valued. At any given time, all able-bodied adults were expected to work, even when they did not feel well. We all actually pulled double duty: Working outside the home and working in the large family garden. My siblings and I would help plant, "pull weeds," and harvest our annual bounty. My grandmother, for example, worked early in the morning in our garden before she and mother would leave for work at a manufacturing plant. Even when my aunts and uncle would move home, they also worked. Among the many family discussions, my mother talked about how at work "Whites" preferred and treated "light skinned" Blacks differently. As a light skinned African American, she not only spoke from experience, but also clearly benefited from this reality in her daily work environment. Family, therefore, is a place where you experienced unconditional acceptance and were taught the subties of your social world. Here, I learned the value of working to make a living, responsibility to the family, and how "shades of color" affected some White people's response and how certain Black people traded on this reality.

Like many youngsters, I became interested in baseball. My older brother and I walked to the Black side of town to play baseball. There, Richard Wood with the help of other Black men organized a little league program for Black youths in the mid 1970s on a rocky field. Years later, he explained the program was needed because the White community refused to allow Black children to play in the local "White" league. Black and White businesses in the town would (or could) only sponsor a number of uniforms that resulted in multiple sponsors for the same team. He was committed to bringing organized baseball, and other community activities, to Black children in the community.

The town shortly sponsored an integrated (i.e., gender and race) little league program and built a new field on the Black side of town. During that initial year, most of the teams were either predominately Black or predominately White, with the exception of one all White team. The season, however, came to an abrupt end after a fight started in the park between two men–one Black and one White–after a Black coach dared to respond to a White lady in the stands after she had yelled a string of insulting remarks toward him. After the city's park and recreation director broke up the fight, in a moment's notice he called off the activities for the remainder of the season. As kids, we were devastated! This experience demonstrated that racial tension remained ever present, right under the community's surface. The efforts of Mr. Wood demonstrated that when local governmental institutions fail to take the lead on unpopular ideas, conscious people can often lead government action.

I started my formal education in 1971. My teachers, Mrs. Thrash and Crocker, a Black and White teacher, respectively, provided my first formal instruction. Later, I learned that the Black teacher was in fact a teacher's aide. The other students were really not an interest to me, as the race of my peers was not an issue. At home, my mother was always reading the newspaper, watching the news, and involved in the church, when she was not working to support the family. I was always fascinated by her interest in the variety of media outlets. So, I began to read the newspaper and watch the news regularly, hoping to find out what was so interesting. The "Watergate hearings," in fact, were among my earliest television images, though at that time, I did not have the vaguest awareness of the national significance of the events unfolding before me on the floor of the living room in the home house.

Unknown to me at the time, my class was among the town's first student cohorts that began their formal education in a fully de-segregated setting. The one thing that always bothered me in primary school was: Why are most of the 'special education' kids Black? Elementary school introduced me to the educational practice of "tracking." This process "reportedly" involved placing students in groups by different "ability levels." Therefore, in fifth grade you were assigned to group A, B, or C. Among the kids, we talked about these groups as the "dumb," "average," and "smart" group, respectively. The racial compositions of these groups were distinct. Group A was almost all Black. It had one or two White kids, who were obviously from poor families. Group B was almost evenly divided with Black and White students. Group C was almost all White. It had one or two Black kids, whose parents were educators or middle class. These observations had me wondering: Are Whites smarter?

Nonetheless, I experienced and witnessed the practice of racial stratification at the institutional levels that attempted to maintain the old racial, social order laid down generations before (Hacker, 1995). Even then, *I knew it was wrong*.

Arguably by design, though arguably fervently denied, I believe only one classmate from that lower track eventually went to college, and he never finished. In terms of timeframe, this occurred over twenty years after *Brown v. Board of Education of 1954*, which theoretically replaced "separate, but equal" as ordered in *Plessey v. Ferguson*. Two generations later, the legacy of Black professionals from previously segregated settings continued to bear fruit in Hogansville. In particular, Black teachers were employed at all levels in the school system and one Black middle school principal.

The presence of Black professionals was a cause for hope. Most were educated at HBCUs, a fact that planted an early seed of possibility. For example, the likes of Rev. (Henry) Johnson, a local A.M.E. minister, history and government teacher, and Morris Brown College alumni stimulated curiosity by his integration of contemporary political issues into lectures. Although a grasp of the textbook content was necessary, he particularly rewarded those who demonstrated knowledge of local and national socio-political issues. The arrival of Edwin Smith, a young African American teacher employed at the high school in the neighborhood whose presence was influential and admired, cannot be underestimated. The importance of a professional role model provided a new and energized self-awareness as well as the potential for greater self-actualization for this teenager. Notably, Mr. Smith has become the county's Superintendent, the first of African descent. After graduating from high school in a class that had almost a fifty-fifty Black/White student composition, I was the only student from the class that initially entered a HBCU. Two others later transferred to Black Colleges; my other African American classmates attended traditional White institutions (TWIs). Some have privately expressed regret for this choice. I did not. Still, most finished their program.

Therefore, my school and community are where I prepared for the broader social world. Here, I learned the value of consuming socio-political information, the influence of positive professional role models, the nature of structural oppression, and that racial tensions rest slightly under our humble community surface. These realities helped to prepare me for the future.

TESTING GROUNDS: OUR ARRIVAL TO COLLEGE

Elaine's Perspective

Because I did not major, or even minor in social studies until late in my college career, and was preparing to teach traditional subjects on a high school level, there was for me little formal learning that shed light on issues of diversity and race. However, at Howard University, our faculty included some of the most renowned luminaries in Negro academia: E. Ernest Just, a renowned scientist who had taught my father and who my father insisted had come closer to producing life in his research than any other in his field; Alain Locke, Charles Wesley, E. Franklin Frazier, Sterlng Brown, Rayford Logan, Eric Williams, and, of course, the famed Howard Thurman.

These men shared their ideas and work at programs on the campus that inspired us. In particular Howard Thurman's ideas stretched my considerations of career choice. At the same time, we were becoming aware of ferment in the city of Washington, D.C. over its rigid segregation policies. I remember particularly the picketing of the People's Drugstore chain which was being well patronized by Blacks. While we did not know it, these activities were early rumblings of the Civil Rights Movement.

Upon graduation, I received a Lucy Moten Fellowship, intended for study abroad; however, because of the war, I was forced to choose study and travel in the U.S. I attended the Lisle Fellowship, a Quaker work camp on Lookout Mountain, Colorado, which became a transformative experience for me. The lectures by well-known academic scholars on philosophy, citizenship participation, responsibility, and spirituality came alive as we applied their principles in our weekend work deputations to the communities surrounding our campsite. We were assigned in teams to meet a variety of needs on farms, in churches, and in social and local government agencies. This is where I learned of migrant farm workers, was shocked at the squalor in which they were forced to live, and saw the deep depression of the Japanese families who had been driven from their homes, mostly in California, and held in internment camps. We led group recreation, taught Sunday school, and even preached sermons in these oppressed communities about which I had heard nothing back East.

The most significant experience was our participation in the Fellowship of Reconciliation (F.O.R.) Conference in Denver. We helped gather data for the workshops the F.O.R. was planning on citizen action to end discrimination, and then were allowed to participate in the workshops themselves. I chose to picket a theatre known to be discriminating against Negroes and Mexicans, was arrested and in jail for several hours. It was the hearing conducted to clear us picketers of charges that was so unforgettable to me. Many citizens articulated their outrage at our arrest, since Colorado had a civil rights law, and we were merely calling attention to its violation. These citizens demanded that the mayor, the police department, and all of the establishments who had been violating the law cease immediately. The passion of these citizens was inspirational and astounding as were the editorials in the Rocky Mountain News. Ironically, I have only realized recently upon finding the program of that Fellowship of Reconciliation conference conducted 64 years ago that it was billed as a "WORKSHOP IN NON VIOLENT ACTION." As we know, the F.O.R. was the forerunner of Congress of Racial Equality (C.O.R.E.), which means that that workshop was a true prelude to the Civil Rights Movement.

In graduate study at the New York School (of Social Work), now Columbia University School of Social Work, my Lisle experience proved to be an interesting foundation for all I was learning. I was exposed to luminaries in the field including Gordon Hamilton, Fern Lowry, Dorothy Hutchinson, Lucille Austin, and Clarence King. However there was very little attention to diversity and race, except for the famous Dollard and Davis Studies, which were pioneering qualitative research studies on the Negro experience.

For my masters' thesis I chose to study the significance of being Negro as seen through parental handling of minority group status. I had been warned that choosing a topic such as this was hazardous since there was so little literature support and faculty would be unfamiliar with the topic. This proved to be true so that I finished my second year of training without completing the thesis. Two years later, after the birth of my first child, my husband, a psychiatrist, helped me to complete it. I was disappointed with the product which seemed vastly less significant than I had planned it to be.

June's Perspective

Attending Spelman College was not my dream, but rather, my mother's. A smart, attractive young woman, she was unable to attend a private school so she went to Florida Agricultural and Mechanical University (formerly Florida A & M College) on a Sojourner Truth Scholarship and as anticipated, excelled. (Sojourner was the brave old slave woman who guided hundreds of fellow slaves to freedom via the Underground Railway.) Spelman was a small college, but located in the gateway to the South or rather, the new South, Atlanta, Georgia. We had spent time in Atlanta, where a paternal Aunt, who was active in the Civil Rights Movement, lived. However, I think my "real" understanding of Atlanta came from reading Margaret Mitchell's best selling book "Gone with the Wind." As an aside, my sister next in line would join me as a child quietly reciting a famous sentence from Rhett Butler to Scarlet O'Hara as she bemoaned his leaving her: "Frankly my dear, I don't give a damn." Of course, neither our parents, Pa'pa, nor household helper ever heard us. One day, one beloved Aunt did. She promised not to tell. Still alive and in her late nineties, she was always held in high esteem since the days I helped her teach and watch for polecats in the back seat of our Ford. What I think this demonstrates is the dominance of structure, pride, and discipline in most Black families (lower, middle, and upper middle class). It is a far cry from today's anti-intellectualism epitomized by rap, misogynist lyrics where women are considered as "bitches" and men "dogs," and many youth never hear correct or "proper" English even uttered. The declining influence of the Black church, a great, important, independent, and influential institution, is also a part of this phenomenon. There were several White professors at Spelman, which represented a new experience for me. Although we had White neighbors and business colleagues in the rural South, there was never a professor or other professionals (i.e., physician, dentist). There were outstanding Black professors just as there had been in my elementary and high schools. These were Professors of my mother's level of intellect and mastery, who could not move into other arenas because of Jim Crow: Professors Marguerite Curry (history), Norman Rates (theology), Lois Moreland (a favorite because of her youth, determination, academic excellence and the confidence she exhibited), and White professors, and one in particular, Howard Zinn (social science), the nationally known historian and author of the best selling *People's History of America* who was my advisor.

These professors, Black and White, encouraged us to excel, though many of us did not always listen. Drs. Moreland and Zinn provided leadership and guidance to young women, several of whom were inclined toward changing the opportunity structure and joining the movement for more open defiance of a segregated system that exploited Blacks and many poor Whites (who likely identified with the ruling structure, and thereby against Blacks). This sentiment had been fermenting and simmering for so very long in many Southern Black churches, where congregations were tired of waiting for the Lord *alone* to make changes for human and communal betterment. For example, the Garys were long time members of Mount Zion African Methodist Episcopal (A.M.E.) Church in Ocala, Florida where learned ministers, Sunday school super-intendents, and teachers reminded us that Richard Allen (founder of the A.M.E. church) led a walkout from the Methodist church in Philadel-phia, where Colored people were seated only in a segregated section. The middle passage along with examples of slave health care and 19th and 20th century quality of life indicators (i.e., housing, education, business) were ever in front of the congregation. Also, the need to pa-tronize Black businesses and own your homes and farms were subjects emphasized.

Dean Whitney Young of the Atlanta University School of Social Work and first President of the National Association of Social Workers (NASW) to be of African descent also provided leadership to the stu-dents from the Atlanta University Center (Clark, Morehouse, Morris Brown, Interdominational Theological Center, and Spelman Colleges, and Atlanta University, the graduate school) and was instrumental along with his wife, a Spelman professor, in recruiting me to the social work profession. In all of my early years, I assumed that I would study and later practice law.

The Spelman College campus leader of the Student Coordinating Movement was Marion Wright (now Marion Wright Edelman, founder and president of the Children's Defense Fund). There were others, and I did not give joining this brave group of students who were planning the participation in sit-ins and other protest a second thought. I joined up. No doubt, my parents assumed that if there were ever a student protest for rights, their children would be counted among the participants. We were. Proudly so. Some of my Spelman schoolmates cited reasons such as potential lost of parents' employment, "unwillingness to miss class," and fear (after all, my generation and proceeding ones had sat-in the back of the bus all of our lives, assuming towns and rural areas even had buses. My town did not).

Getting arrested, being hauled off in a paddy wagon are unforgettable, but clearly important moments. Now, I think: So what, if we integrated hot dog and hamburger counters, if so many cannot afford to even pur-chase that cheap unhealthy food. The issue then was about rights, and it remains so today, including the right to a basic, adequate education, and, just as importantly, health care, housing, and employment.

In professional school at Atlanta University, I had a major "eye-opener." Completing an aspect of a group research thesis, which was not at my placement, The Metropolitan Youth Commission Project, but at the Department of Public Welfare, St. Louis, Missouri, where there were sufficient data, I learned that Black social workers were not permitted to serve White clients, whereas White social workers could serve clients regardless of race. I expected and was aware of blatant discrimination in social work practice in Georgia and the deep South, but in St. Louis? After all, that city was the site of the 1857 Dread Scott Decision. Had the people learned anything about social rights?

My doctoral education was at the distinguished Heller School, Brandeis University. Only a few women had completed their course of study when I entered as a young woman in the late 1960s and finished quite quickly in two and a half years. Andrew Billingsely and Charlotte Dunmore, were role models and, more critical, evidence that you could get through the program. Faculty and fellow students were mostly very supportive, and especially the Dean, Charles I. Schottland. To my knowledge, the school, however, has been slow to develop a diverse faculty and staff although, arguably, it did a fine job in graduating a diverse group of competent, committed, individuals who have carried significant leadership roles in the profession. What is clear is that many faculties will not easily share power, although they might well proffer otherwise regarding expectations of external organizations.

My first full time teaching position was at the Ohio State University (OSU). That institution appeared particularly reactionary after the Brandeis experience, which had been a hotbed of intellectual ideas and ferment and political activism. There was ferment over the Vietnam War throughout the campus, and all were mindful of that sad day at Kent State University, where the Ohio National Guard killed college students who were protesting the war. Students and professors debated the war, intensely, with fervor and deep concern about the country's future. President Nixon brought some closure to the war in time, but later, the country was consumed with Watergate. Both Vietnam and Watergate became defining moments in the country and the latter brought the country to a low level of self-respect. What I remember most about OSU was the perception of unequal financial rewards for women who held similar educational credentials and worked as hard as men. I helped organize a group to examine this issue. I was convinced that the perception was true, as did most (if not all) of the other women. The prevailing attitude was not "comparable worth." Before entering OSU, I was employed briefly at Boston University in the Afro-American Studies program working under an outstanding sociologist–African Scholar, a graduate of Smith College and Harvard University. Outspoken, exquisite, and brilliant,

Professor Adelaide Cromwell was one of the first colleagues to indicate that I had a serious interest in research and encouraged me in that direction. She was a solid role model, who has just recently published a book in 2007 on how her family moved from slave status to free Black.

Tony's Perspective

Arriving at Grambling State University helped me in different ways. As a first generation college student, the familiarity of people (i.e., faculty, staff, students) that looked like me made the social transition more comforting and provided cultural affirmation at this important junction in my development. It also was the first time that I had attended a predominately-Black institution with exception of my local church, Hill Chapel United Methodist. Here, Black people served in every capacity from cafeteria workers, accountants, nurses, program managers, professors, departmental heads and deans, and even President of the institution. This reality spoke to me literally as I remember Dr. Grace Tatem, a Social Work Professor saying, "I have to prepare you students to replace me." These were important words for a young social work student to hear as it told me I could also become a college professor one day. In contrast, after I openly stated in one class my plans to pursue a PhD, the White faculty member openly laughed. This class of all Black students looked on, but no one found it funny, and she laughed alone. Although her laughter cut deeply, and I felt hurt, I would not be deterred.

In the meantime, my early political awakening began to get traction. Although my home and community of origin had nurtured the early interest in socio-political issues, college became a place to exercise these passions. Here, I first became involved in voter registration efforts as Rev. Jesse Jackson's first presidential run energized many African American youths all across the country. Among the many themes echoed by student organizers, voting privileges won by previous generations had to be respected, utilized, and exercised. We did just that. In fact, Grambling's college chapter of the National Association for the Advancement of Colored People (NAACP) at that time was the largest in the nation. This was nurtured as students would hear the likes of current and former state and national governmental leaders and scholars.

Still, the gubernatorial run in Louisiana of State Representative David Dukes (Republican), a former Grand Wizard of the Ku Klux Klan and founding President of the National Association for the Advancement of White People, compelled many African American students to mobilize politically. I was a part of this wave. In response, the voter registration rate of African Americans in Louisiana reportedly approached 90 percent. We knew that we had to hold back race-bating politics that sought to undermine the political gains fought for by our predecessors. The School of Social Work's first Dean, Dr. William Pollard (1978) wrote a book entitled, *A Study of Black Self-Help*, which was a required reading. This book chronicled how Southern Blacks mobilized their limited resources to address the needs of their communities. We knew as young social work and Black college students in general that this was our moment. We had an obligation to *stand up* and let our voices be heard at the voting box.

Upon entering my social work field placement, unlike many of my colleagues before me, I could serve all clients. While I had always known that there were poor White people, I never really knew just how poor some were. My field placement in Monroe, Louisiana had me serving some clients from the Mississippi Delta region. There, I met Black and White consumers of mental health and substance abuse services who shared with me a level of poverty that I never knew existed in America. In fact, one report referred to it as "third world in America." From this experience, I came away with the new realization that abject poverty among White people was hidden. From these consumers, I sensed that they feared that they represented a "shame" among other White folks. Then, I wondered, are poor Blacks seen in the same way among other middle and upper class Blacks?

My doctoral education was at the University of Pittsburgh's School of Social Work. My choice for this school was driven by it's reputation, history, faculty, and national status among the nation's most esteemed Schools of Social Work. Dean David Epperson, one of the nation's longest serving Social Work Deans, embodied a confidence and participatory leadership style that provided a role model for anyone with an interest in educational leadership for the future. The fact that he was African American was only an added plus for me. He often reminded his students and others that he stood on the shoulders of many others. I was proud to have served as his graduate administrative assistant before he retired, because it afforded me the opportunity to learn by asking questions, watching, and listening. I view myself as one of many standing on his knowledgeable and broad shoulders.

I later learned that my cohort's entry into the program came with some fanfare. This cohort of nine doctoral students included three African American males. The fact that a third of the class was composed of African American males was highly unusual for most doctoral programs. For me, it was both comforting and empowering to know that I had colleagues with common ancestry and possible experiences. Despite differences in age, marital life stage (and status), and region of origin, we shared common perspectives and believed in many similar ideals. Someone challenged the qualifications of the cohort, and the objective data reaffirmed that the school had accepted the best qualified candidates. This led me to wonder, whether the proportion of African Americans was the basis of this challenge? We each finished. However, the support provided from within and outside of the group was an important factor for successful, timely completion.

During our studies at Pittsburgh, one racial incident was decidedly pronounced. Here, we were confronted with gross, racially insensitive comments from a faculty member in a seminar session who disparaged Black men in general. Despite the fact that the majority of students in the seminar were African American, the professor seemed oblivious to the depth of this verbal assault. We glanced at each other for a brief moment. Then, I spoke up by challenging the validity of the comments and dismissing his remarks as stereotypically rooted in a bygone age. Others agreed. This professor had held several major leadership positions in the profession and was well respected as a thoughtful, scholarly colleague; yet, sadly he never understood his own prejudice.

PRACTICE AND TEACHING EXPERIENCES

Elaine's Perspective

My professional experience began as a psychiatric social worker in a child guidance clinic in a large, well known teaching hospital. While it provided excellent training in traditional mental health practice, there was no attention to diversity and race. When the Civil Rights Movement began heating up, I felt compelled to take my skills to work in the Black community. Housed there was a small preschool psychiatric clinic which was world renowned, had trained seventy five percent of the pre-school child psychiatrists in the country, was psychoanalytically based and staffed by outstanding, internationally recognized clinicians and researchers. It had largely excluded neighborhood people from its caseload, but was now committed to serving the local population. Becoming chief social worker there, I learned firsthand how issues of race and racism can undermine service to poor and oppressed populations, creating enigmas, inconsistencies and complexities that are entrapping and stressful. I learned about the chaos and stress that ensues when experts attempt to offer services to a population they do not understand and become threatened. When their lack of expertise is challenged, they are unable to alter their power position as experts who inappropriately diagnose, treat, and do research, and cannot easily assume the necessary position of listener, learner or student. Elsewhere I have described in some detail this experience that opened my eyes to how persons in power behave when that power is threatened and/or must be shared, and how persons with less power operate to empower themselves and acquire power.

I believe that it was the combination of sound clinical training and work in excellent settings combined with a later move to academia that facilitated my survival. Being able to use theory to conceptualize the confusion, conflict, and stress I had found in practice became a therapeutic act and an unexpected source of liberation. Joining the faculty of a school of social work required me to develop a high level of theory mastery in order to teach human behavior, personality development, family therapy theory, systems functioning, and advanced practice and gave me the tools needed to conceptualize what I had learned and would learn. Grounding my rich though stressful experiences in theory and even developing concepts of my own to explain the dynamics in which I had been trapped, led to writing and publishing and a palpable sense of control over the overwhelming sadness, confusion, pain, and sense of powerlessness I had internalized during those last very stressful years of practice.

I have been particularly dedicated to understanding and conceptualizing the ways in which the systemic operation of difference and power in human functioning (1) operate to maintain racism, sexism, classism, homophobia, discrimination and injustice, (2) in turn, influence individual, family, group and community processes, and (3) are also key in our work. An opportunity to conduct research among the Yoruba in Nigeria shed light on how these dynamics have operated during the enslavement-and-after process for African Americans causing them to sustain enormous losses by fragmenting their ethnic fabric and subjecting them to repeated transgenerational traumas. Researching my own family allowed me to apply that understanding of the operation of difference and power as they have affected the African American experience to my own family. This genealogical sojourn has been transformative in my life. Teaching and writing about diversity thus became a personal mental health issue for me and central in my journey to become a practitioner, educator, consultant, and author. But although the way was marked often by bewilderment, frustration, and stress, it has also brought enormous rewards.

June's Perspective

Boston College was a terrific experience. Working with and for a Jesuit institution and leadership was both personally and professionally rewarding. The emphasis on caring for the total person as a driving force in the intellectual, spiritual, and moral development of students was genuine and well implemented via teaching, research, and local field instructional and international experiences. There were questions relative to diversity, gender, and race, but these were dealt with under the leadership of first rate minds, starting with the President J. Donald Monan, S.J. (Society of Jesus) and a host of Jesuit academic Vice Presidents. These questions, especially regarding gender and the role of women, were long standing—as they are in other faith communities.

The Graduate School of Social Work (GSSW) flourished in no small part because of the President and other top executives' commitment coupled with the determination for excellence and high professional status exhibited by faculty and the alumni board. I am not implying that there were not tensions related to diversity nor that some groups felt marginalized. What I can say is that in comparison to other Schools of Social Work where I have been employed and visited for re-accreditation or consultation, the drive for social and economic justice was less controversial and egregious. This might well be attributed to the experience of historical rejection, discrimination, and servitude that challenged Catholics in Boston. After all, one reason that the GSSW was founded was to open up greater opportunities for the Irish and other immigrant groups who faced discrimination at the one existing School of Social Work in Boston. In fact, the School's founder, Fr. Walther McGuinn, S.J., hired a distinguished, classy, well educated Protestant woman from New York City to open up the brahmin social agencies. She exceeded, and faculty who remembered her initiative recall it being far from easy. Dorothy Book is a revered name at Boston College GSSW—the institution where I served as dean and professor for twenty four years.

June's and Tony's Current Perspectives

Our experiences at UGA are still evolving. Nonetheless, there are several activities that have been a part of our professional engagement for a period of time that warrant reflection. The population of the State of Georgia is almost a third African-American and their population at the flagship university is less than 7 percent; for Black males it is slightly over 2 percent. For all students of color, the numbers lag their representation. Severely so. The central administration building is Holmes-Hunter, named in honor of the brave students who put a face on the fight for desegregation, the late Hamilton Holmes, M.D. and Charlene Hunter-Gault, journalist/Johannesburg CNN Bureau Chief, South Africa. The question is how and to what extent diversity is acknowledged. The current President and Provost have certainly spoken to and acted on the need for greater representation of the State's population in administrative appointments, faculty, and the distribution of the university's honors and symbols. However, no one would argue that the legacy is still nearly "lily white." The three honorary degrees awarded to African Americans were all done under the current administrative leadership. There are other symbols that continue to reflect a time that many thought had "gone with the wind."

An issue often articulated is how to educate the emerging Hispanic population and, in the School of Social Work, prepare a cadre of competent professionals for the herculean professional iniatives with this needful group. What is missing, overlooked, and/or ignored is how can and will an institution that has not been sufficiently dedicated, let alone successful, in servicing another needful constituency that has been on the scene since the founding of the state and helped build its physical and economic structures and resources prepare to serve Hispanics? In the absence of a history and tradition of service to a disparate African American population, is it reasonable to assume success in work with another population that brings even greater cultural/language diversity and barriers? A positive outcome would be embraced!

Political dynamics (via voting rights and activities) will drive some change. But, has the overall university faculty and staff, grown accustomed to a "private" environment? Can the ideology and symbols that promote inclusion be incorporated in sufficient timeliness? Much goodwill does exist and should promote an ongoing climate of positive change for the betterment of the state's workforce.

DISCUSSION

Each author, though decades apart, experienced similar challenges because of race (more than gender). The early days of change oriented ferment, commencing with her experience in a drug store, were noted by Elaine, who grew up in a middle class environment. June grew up on a farm with only a few nearby neighbors, who were mostly White. All got along, though their lives were separate. She participated in the 1960s sit-ins, which were tactics used by college students to press for greater inclusion, a goal that corresponded with the larger Civil Rights Movement identified more broadly with Rosa Parks and Martin Luther King. Tony reaped some of the anticipated benefits of the Civil Rights Movement as a child beginning with a de-segregated school experience. Although he lived his early life on the predominately "White" side of town, his family's social reference group was clearly Black, and he was (and is) confronted with lingering residue from the Jim Crow age.

Another commonality was that all three attended HBCUs, those institutions that were established to accept Black students. The role of HBCUs is the mission of successfully producing educated talented Blacks who would take their place in American society. These institutions prepared the first African American on the Supreme Court, many leading professionals and politicians. Their role is still critical even though academic institutions, who for the most part denied admissions to Blacks until the later part of the 20th century, "voice" interest in recruiting them today.

Finally, an awareness of privileges and barriers related to shades of "blackness" is apparent. The three authors had a parent who helped their family because of employment and business advantages that accrued to those with light skin. For this reason, they recognize the subtlety of within group privilege afforded to members of their family, but also are particularly aware of the impact on the lives of the Black masses.

The three of us conclude that it was easier to fight the ideology voiced by such Southern Governors as George Wallace, Herman Talmadge, Lester Maddox, Oval Fabus, state representative and gubernatorial candidate David Dukes, and Bull Connor, the infamous police chief, all dedicated segregationist, than it is to fight the current social/economic disparities and imbalances led by multi-national corporations (who pulled out of local communities and out sourced labor), quiet, subtle racism (as opposed to blatant), Black intra-group apathy, anti-intellectualism, family discontinuity and challenges, hopelessness and undoubtedly the new slave system, drugs.

IMPLICATIONS FOR DIVERSITY AND SOCIAL JUSTICE

No one recalls social work rushing to acknowledge diversity and social economic justice, let alone to embrace it. The CSWE had a struggle on its hand. The movement to downplay poverty and the poor was very much related to the desire to distance the profession from service to people of color (after all poor and color are so very closely correlated). Many faculty members did and continue to resist diversity and co-relative power sharing, and gender and racial/ethnic parity. The question of faculty autonomy, and even academic freedom were messages heard, but in effect, were they not messages to stonewall? Admitting new groups into the academy means some old faces will not be at the table in numbers seen in decades past. But, there is a struggle: White men will give little, but they will not give it up–without a push. The current question: Will White women mimic their husbands, brothers, fathers, and sons or will they share power and privilege with women and men of color?

Even though the profession's history is not stellar, it is not all reactionary or negative. More recently, it has emphasized the need for structural change, socio-political parity, and social justice. The question remains whether it can or will exercise sufficient leadership, critical thinking, and scholarship to get the job done. We have hope and yes, social work is still the country's most open profession.

REFERENCES

Author. (2006). Legacy: Ollie and Homer Gary. *Ocala Charity Register*, p. 96.

Billingsely, A. (1968). *Black families in White America.* Englewood Cliffs, NJ. Prentice Hall.

Billingsley, A. (1992). *Climbing Jacob's ladder: The enduring legacy of African-American families.* New York: Simon & Schuster.

Byrant, M. (2007). Simpler times: Blacks recall booming business in Ocala. *Star-Banner, May 9.* [Electronic version] Retrieved on August 27, 2007 (www.ocala.com).

Cromwell, A. (2007). Unveiled voices, unvarnished memories: The Cromwell family in slavery and segregation, 1692-1972. Columbia, MO: University of Missouri Press.

Daniels, M. (2001). *Horace T. Ward: Desegregation of the University of Georgia, civil rights advocacy, and jurisprudence,* Atlanta, GA: Clark Atlanta University Press.

DuBois, W. E. B. (1903, 1999). The souls of Black folk. H. L. Gates, Jr. and T. H. Oliver (Eds). New York: W.W. Norton Company.

Hacker, A. (1995). *Two nations: Black and White, separate, hostile, unequal.* New York: Ballantine Book.

Hopps, J. G. (2006). *Still striving: Challenges for board of trustees of historically black college*. Atlanta, GA: Southern Education Foundation.

Hopps, J. G., Tourse, R. W. C., & Christian, O. (2002). From problems to personal resilience: Challenges and opportunities 91/2 in practice with African American youth. *Journal of Ethnic & Cultural Diversity in Social Work, 11 (1/2)*, 55-77.

Lincoln, C. E. & Mamiya, L. H. (1990). *The Black church in the African American experience*. Durham, N.C.: Duke University Press.

Lefever, H. G. (2005). *Undaunted by the fight: Spelman College and the Civil Rights Movement, 1957-1967*. Macon: Mercer University Press.

Logan, S. M. L. (1990). Diversity among black families: Assessing structure and function. In S. M. L. Logan, E. M. Freeman, & R. G. McRoy (Eds.). *Social work practice with Black families: A culturally specific perspective*, pp. 73-96. White Plain, NY: Longman.

Lowe, T. B. & Hopps, J. G. (2007). African American's response to their social environment: A macro perspective. In L. See (Ed.). *An African American Perspectives in Human Behavior in the Social Environment* (2nd ed.). New York: Haworth Press, Inc.

Martin, E. & Martin, J. (1985). *The helping tradition in the Black family and community*. Silver Spring, MD: National Association of Social Workers.

McRoy, R. G. (1990). A historical overview of the black families. In S. M. L. Logan, E. M. Freeman, & R. G. McRoy (Eds.). *Social work practice with Black families: A culturally specific perspective*. White Plain, NY: Longman.

Moynihan, D. P. (1965). *The Negro family: The case for national action*. Washington, DC: U.S. Government Printing Office.

Pollard, W. (1978). *A study of Black self-help*. San Francisco: R & E Research Associates.

Saleeby, D. (2002). *The strengths perspective in social work practice* (3rd ed.). Boston: Turner: Allyn & Bacon.

Sitkoff, H. (1993). *The struggle for Black equality 1954-1992* (Revised ed.). New York: The Noonday Press.

Stewart, J. C. (1996). *1001 history things everyone should know about African Americans history*. New York: Doubleday.

Young, W. M., Jr. (1964). *To be equal*. New York: McGraw-Hill.

Index